Love
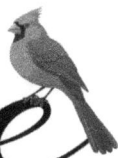
BEYOND

DAWN LOHR

Love
BEYOND

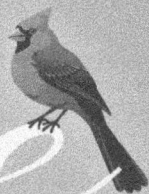

A MOTHER'S HEART,
A SON'S COURAGEOUS BATTLE

Advantage | Books

Published by Advantage Books, Charleston, South Carolina.
An imprint of Advantage Media.

ADVANTAGE is a registered trademark, and the Advantage colophon is a trademark of Advantage Media Group, Inc.

Printed in the United States of America.

10 9 8 7 6 5 4 3 2 1

ISBN: 979-8-89188-032-0 (Hardcover)
ISBN: 979-8-89188-033-7 (eBook)

Library of Congress Control Number: 2025910732

Cover design by Megan Elger.
Front flap illustration by Seongah Choi.
Layout design by Ruthie Wood.

This publication is designed to provide accurate and authoritative information in regard to the subject matter covered. It is sold with the understanding that the publisher is not engaged in rendering legal, accounting, or other professional services. If legal advice or other expert assistance is required, the services of a competent professional person should be sought.

Advantage Books is an imprint of Advantage Media Group. Advantage Media helps busy entrepreneurs, CEOs, and leaders write and publish a book to grow their business and become the authority in their field. Advantage authors comprise an exclusive community of industry professionals, idea-makers, and thought leaders. For more information go to **advantagemedia.com**.

To my beloved son Jonathan Andrew, you are an inspiration of courage and hope. I know you are at peace now. I will be your voice and honor your life. I miss you, and I know I will see you again. You are and always will be a gift from God. Love, Mom.

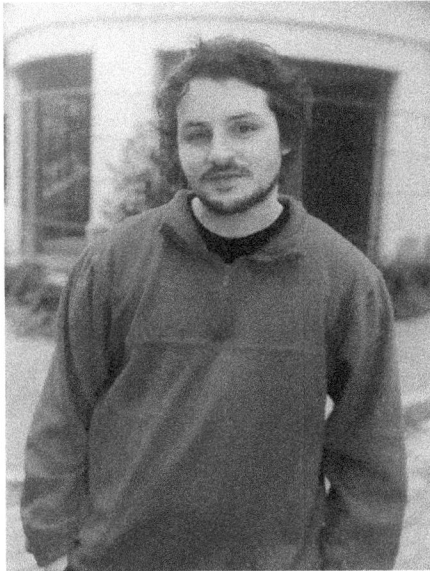

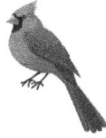

CONTENTS

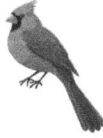

FOREWORD

by Suzanna de Boer,
Editor and Book Coach

When I first began working with Dawn Lohr on her book *Love Beyond*, the story we set out to tell was very different from the one you now hold in your hands. At the time, her beloved son Jonathan was still alive—struggling, yes, but surrounded by support, treatment, and the fierce, unwavering love of his family. There was a flicker of hope. The early drafts of this manuscript reflected that hope: a mother's determined journey to help her son heal, and a young man's brave attempt to navigate the darkness of depression.

Dawn's original vision was a book that might show the path toward recovery. A story of resilience, understanding, and ultimately, triumph over mental illness.

But life, as it so often does, had other plans.

As we continued our work together—editing chapters, deepening character arcs, shaping a narrative both emotionally rich and brutally honest—the unthinkable happened. Jonathan took his own life.

Everything changed.

And yet, Dawn kept writing. Not just for herself, but for every parent who has ever watched their child suffer in silence. For every young person who feels invisible in their pain. For every family walking through the shadows of mental health, feeling unsure, overwhelmed, or alone. She rewrote this book—not to offer a promise that all stories end in recovery but to offer a different kind of hope. The kind that comes through remembrance. Through truth-telling. Through love that continues, even in grief.

Love Beyond is the embodiment of that love. Told in alternating voices between Maria (Dawn's fictionalized version of herself) and Josh (Jonathan), it is a profoundly intimate look inside a family's battle with depression, anxiety, and the heartbreak of suicide. What makes this book extraordinary is not just the depth of pain it chronicles but the courage and clarity with which it does so.

This is not an easy story—but it is a necessary one.

Dawn gives voice to the questions so many parents silently carry: How do I help my child? What did I miss? Could I have done more? And through Jonathan's chapters, she creates space for readers to step inside the lived experience of a teenager who appears to "have it all" but feels lost, unseen, and exhausted beneath the surface.

The authenticity of this book is both its power and its gift. It doesn't shy away from the hard moments—the confusion, the missteps, the fear, the numbing grief—but neither does it abandon us there. Instead, *Love Beyond* leads us, page by page, toward understanding, compassion, and the possibility of healing.

As Dawn's editor and book coach, I witnessed not just the creative process but the emotional fortitude it took to keep going. She didn't have to finish this book. Many wouldn't have. But she chose to honor Jonathan's life by telling the full truth of his story, and in doing so, she has created something enduring—a legacy of love and a lifeline for others.

The courage I witnessed in Dawn was extraordinary. Her decision to keep writing even through the most devastating heartbreak a parent can experience left a lasting impression on me, both personally and professionally. This is a mother who chose to transform pain into purpose. Her vulnerability on the page is matched only by her deep desire to help others feel seen, heard, and less alone. I am endlessly inspired by her and honored to be part of this essential project.

If you are holding this book because you are hurting, know this: You are not alone. If you are a parent, a teacher, a friend, or someone who simply wants to better understand mental health, this book will open your eyes and soften your heart. And if you, like Josh, are fighting a quiet battle no one else can see, may this book remind you how deeply your life matters.

This is not a story with a fairytale ending. But it is a story of extraordinary love. Of presence. Of staying close to those we love, even when they are slipping beyond our reach.

And in that, there is hope—not the fragile kind, dependent on circumstances, but the fierce, enduring kind that lives on in memory, in advocacy, and in every act of love we carry forward. There is hope in the telling. There is hope in the healing. And there is hope in knowing that even the deepest pain can give rise to purpose, connection, and light.

This book is part of that light—and each purchase helps the Jonathan Andrew Foundation make costly therapy treatments available to young adults facing mental health challenges.

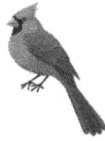

CHAPTER ONE

Simple Days

Josh

"Hey, Josh, what a fantastic save!" Alec yells as he comes toward me.

"Thanks, man," I reply, pulling off my sweat-soaked goalie glove to shake his hand.

"These summer practices are grueling. I'll never get used to the Charleston heat."

"The heat is bad, but the humidity is unbearable." I chuckle, wiping sweat from my forehead with the bottom of my T-shirt.

Alec is my best friend. From kindergarten until high school, he and I have done everything together. Lately, I haven't wanted to hang out with him—*or anybody, for that matter.*

"I haven't seen you all summer. You OK, man?" Alec asks.

"Yeah, just been tired lately," I tell him. It's true, *but it's not the whole truth.*

I'm not myself; I'm moody, sad, and no fun to be around.

"There's a party tonight for Justin's birthday. Hope you can come," Alec says, smiling.

"Thanks for letting me know. I might just chill tonight."

"OK, I'm here if you want to talk about anything." Alec looks concerned as he touches my shoulder.

"Thanks, I really appreciate that." I look down at my untied cleat.

"See you at school," he says as he turns to head to his silver Honda Accord.

I have enjoyed the summer and playing soccer. School starts in a week. Senior year.

I should be excited, but right now I really don't care one way or the other. I think of my mom; she is in "crazy mom mode." I just had my senior pictures taken. Mom loves them, commenting specifically on how my eyes look bright green and how curly my dark hair was that day. She says it makes me look grown-up and like a little boy at the same time. She's already making plans for graduation, asking me where I want to have dinner and making a list of who all will be there. What she doesn't know is that I could care less about graduation dinner; *I just want the year to be over.*

Standing there looking at the soccer field, I remember all the times I've walked onto the field and into the goalie box. I love playing soccer. I've always felt at home on the field. I love being part of a team, and I've found that being a goalie allows me to challenge myself to be my best. My perfect eyesight and fearlessness help me to stop almost every shot. I don't like to boast about myself, but I'm really good in the goalie box. I get a rush when the opponent kicks the ball to score. I've always been confident and strong on the soccer field.

Off the field, I am not.

I did have a concussion in eighth grade that still worries Mom. *But I'm fine.*

Mom goes to all of my games, as she does with all of my siblings—Curt's baseball games, Audra's dance recitals, and AJ's track meets. I was a sophomore on the varsity team when we won playoffs and went on to play in the state championships. Mom cheered me on through the whole tournament. I remember seeing her smile at me from the sidelines. Dad goes when he can, but I've seen him less and less since their divorce. It used to upset me, but not so much anymore.

I reach down to pick up my favorite, worn soccer ball. I trace a faded black pentagon with my thumb. I always feel better after a good soccer game. I smile as I walk to my car.

See, some things still make me smile. Why can't I shake this sad feeling that seems to follow me these days?

I decide to talk to Mom about it when I get home. I'm not sure she will know what to do, but it's worth asking her for help because I know how much she cares for me.

I blast my music on my radio to drown out my thoughts on the drive home.

Pulling into the driveway of my childhood home, I feel sad again and decide against talking to Mom. I walk up the path to our Charleston green front door (which I always thought was black). I head upstairs to take a shower. As I'm getting out of the shower, the phone rings—it's Carrie.

"Hi, uh, how are you?" I ask her nervously, stumbling over my words.

"I'm doing great. How are you?" Carrie asks me.

"I'm OK," I tell her halfheartedly. I've been avoiding her and haven't told her how I'm feeling.

"Would you like to go to the beach with me next Saturday?" she asks.

"Sure, I would love to meet you at the beach. See you then. Bye."

I met Carrie at the beginning of our junior year. She had just moved from Pennsylvania with her family because of her father's new job at Boeing.

She is beautiful. I like her red hair and her green eyes. And I love her big heart. She's so kind to everyone. I honestly don't know what she sees in me. We've been dating for a year now.

I've avoided sharing with her how depressed I am.

"I will enjoy spending time with her," I say to my reflection to convince myself.

I have seen Mom talk to herself in the mirror; maybe this forced positivity will work for me too.

I feel very excited to see Carrie during the drive to the beach. Every time I cross the bridge over the intercoastal waterway, I feel peaceful. The marsh grass, once green, has faded to brown from the scorching summer heat. The low country of South Carolina is always fascinating to me. I see egrets in the marsh water, now at low tide. These white, long-necked birds always remind me of a plastic lawn bird, although Mom says they are very majestic.

As I reach the end of the bridge, I see the tops of the trees—oaks and palms mixed together. Beyond the trees, I see the sparkling blue water of the Atlantic Ocean.

I love seeing the ocean.

I really love living here.

I finally arrive, park, and grab my beach towel. As I cross over the boardwalk to the beach, a family of pelicans flies in a straight line over my head—almost as if they are guiding me. I see Carrie sitting in our favorite spot on Sullivan's Island. There is not a cloud in the sky, and I can feel the summer sun warm my skin.

"Hi, Josh, I'm over here!" Carrie announces to the whole beach as I walk between the dunes and toward her.

She runs right up to me and hugs me.

"I'm really happy to see you," she booms.

"I'm happy to see you too," I say, grinning.

Carrie has planned everything: Chick-fil-A biscuits and orange juice for breakfast, lunch for later, a soccer ball, and a Frisbee. She even brought a beach chair, sunscreen, and a towel for me too. Sitting next to her with the sun on our faces as we watch the waves is wonderful. We sit in silence after we finish our breakfast, just holding hands. I look down at our hands together—I like seeing our fingers intertwined, and I feel her strength transfer to me.

I know Carrie is happy, and I want to be happy too.

"Last one in is a rotten egg!" Carrie yells, jumping up and running to the water.

"No one says that anymore!" I yell back, following right behind her.

"I do," she says, laughing as she turns around to kiss me.

Every time she kisses me, fireworks explode inside. Simple things like sitting beside her, holding her hand, seeing her smile, and kissing her make me very happy.

I will not have sad thoughts today, I tell myself.

"Thank you!" I shout out to her as the waves crash around us.

Carrie doesn't ask what for; she just smiles at me.

We spend all day at the beach. I'm thankful Carrie doesn't mention our senior year or going off to college. She always knows the right thing to say or not to say.

When the day is over, we pack everything up, and I help Carrie carry it to her car.

I didn't want the day to end.

"Want to go see that new James Bond movie on Friday night with me?" Carrie asks.

"Yes, I can pick you up," I tell her.

I know Carrie is very independent, but Mom always wants me to be a gentleman.

She stops to look at me, brushing the strands of her auburn hair that fell out of her ponytail away from her eyes. I really look at her; she is so beautiful. I feel like the luckiest guy in the world. I want her to know she makes me feel that way, but I let my nerves stop me.

"Bye, Josh, see you Friday," she whispers after I kiss her. She starts walking back to her car.

"Carrie." Hearing my voice, she turns around. "Thank you for a wonderful day."

"You're so welcome," she says with a smile.

I want every day to be like today.

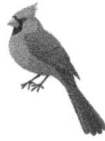

CHAPTER TWO

Hiding Feelings

Maria

Another summer is over, and the kids will start a new school year. It's Josh's senior year.

Josh has been very reserved and kept to himself lately. He has not seen his friends or Carrie all summer. He didn't even come down for dinner tonight. His dad, Aaron, and I have always encouraged our children to talk to us about anything. Since we divorced two years ago, Josh has come to us less and less.

Josh is my second son. He is friends with everyone, and he's always been very happy. Curt, my oldest son, is the shy, reserved, and sometimes moody one. Audra has always been confident and strong; she has to be, with three brothers. My youngest son, AJ, is so funny and full of energy. While they are all different in wonderful ways, Josh's demeanor seems particularly unusual these days.

I created my first list for his senior year: select best senior pictures, order cap and gown, remind Josh of college application deadlines, and submit form for financial aid. This is the first time I'm doing all of the senior stuff on my own, as Aaron helped with Curt's senior year. Of course, as their dad, he still helps with some of the school things. However, the majority of it falls on me.

I decide that I'll do more of this later. Since I have a day off, I really want to enjoy this beautiful summer afternoon. I head upstairs in search of my pannier, sunscreen, and towel. I put on my favorite red bikini and black cover-up. Grabbing my flip-flops and beach chair, I get in my black SUV and head to the beach.

I'm so happy to have my favorite stretch of beach all to myself. Seeing the sun shining on the bright blue ocean brings back so many wonderful memories of my childhood with my brother and parents on the beach in Ocean City, Maryland.

Sitting on the beach, I suddenly remember the summer before my senior year. My parents had just signed the final papers for their divorce. I spent most of the summer working and with my friends, so I didn't have to be in my childhood home that my dad no longer lived in. It still makes me sad to think about my parents' divorce.

I have mastered the art of keeping myself busy as a way of avoiding my feelings. After my parents split, I chose a college farther away from the small, single-stoplight town that I grew up in. I attended Loyola University in Baltimore, Maryland. Smiling, I recall my roommates, who are still my great friends. I want my children to have wonderful college experiences and great friends for life too. Now that Aaron and I are separated, I realize that our children are likely to be sad too.

I want our children to have better ways to express their feelings than the ways I have adopted.

My mind has been all over the place, thinking about my past a lot the last three days. I notice a ghost crab coming out of a hole in the sand to explore the beach.

Closing my eyes, I feel the sun on my face. *I do love the beach.* I feel at peace here.

Oh no—it's 7:00 a.m. I need to hurry, or I'll be late for work. *As my feet hit the floor, I recall that I have a three-day weekend, and it's only Saturday.*

Climbing back into bed, I pull the covers over my head to block the sun peeping through the bedroom windows. Blackout shades would have been a great investment, but money is tight following the divorce.

Ugh, I can't go back to sleep.

My king-sized sleigh bed is very comfortable, so I decide to just lie here. The fan above is whirring around and around, just like the thoughts in my head.

I'm really worried about Josh.

I say a quick prayer. "God, I really don't know how to help Josh. He doesn't seem to be himself these days. Please help him."

I can't shake the feeling that something is very wrong. Tears fill my eyes at the thought that something is hurting my son.

I know the divorce has been tough on all my kids. I did not want them to experience the same pain that I did with my parents' divorce.

I will talk to Josh today.

I pull my long, dark hair into a ponytail. Putting on my yoga pants and my favorite hot-pink top, I start a yoga YouTube video to move my body and clear my mind.

Drying off after my post-workout shower, I smile.

"You still got it, even as a single mom of four," I tell my reflection.

I smell the coffee beckoning me downstairs.

As I'm enjoying my first sip of my favorite French coffee, I decide that I'm going to make Josh's favorite meal for dinner. It will just be him and me tonight. Curt is in Europe, traveling with his high school friends, Audra is visiting friends in the North Carolina mountains, and AJ is with his dad for the weekend. This will give Josh and me some quality time to catch up over dinner when he gets back from his beach day with Carrie.

Pulling out my old cookbook, I start looking for Grandma's lasagna recipe. I will make homemade sauce for him too. The memory of Josh with sauce all over his little face as a baby brings tears to my eyes. I love to cook for my kids.

Josh will be graduating soon, and he will be out on his own. I know he's a young man, but I still see him as my little boy. *I will make the most of this year with him.*

I relax on the back porch with a glass of fresh-brewed, unsweetened iced tea. I cannot drink the syrupy, sweet tea that Southerners love. I check on my sauce throughout the afternoon between chapters of the latest book I'm reading.

I finish layering the lasagna noodles, ricotta cheese mixture, and sauce in the pan. As I put the pan in the oven, Josh walks in the front door. He looks wonderful. The sun-kissed color of his skin and the smile on his face are both radiant.

"How was your day?" I ask, knowing the answer already.

"It was fantastic!" he exclaims. "It smells great in here. I'm going to shower, and then I will be down to eat."

I let out a sigh; I had been holding my breath. I feel relieved, seeing Josh so happy.

I return to the back porch while the lasagna bakes in the oven. As I pick up my book again, the phone rings.

"Oh, hi, Janet. So great to hear from you."

"Maria, how is Josh?" Janet asks. "The boys have not seen much of each other lately. Can we all get together?"

"I believe he's doing well. He spent the day at the beach with Carrie. He looked so happy coming home just now. I agree that he and Alec have spent less time together; I will encourage Josh to hang out more. I would love to have you both to dinner soon. Talk to you later."

Janet's like a sister to me, and our boys are like brothers. She would do anything for Josh, and I would do anything for Alec. So naturally, Janet has been a little worried about Josh lately. Maybe a dinner would be a good opportunity for them to talk to Josh too. I head back inside and turn off the oven.

"Dinner's ready," I announce, thrilled about the meal I have made for my son. It's nice to be having dinner with just him.

"Wow, Mom, this is delicious!" Josh exclaims after taking his first bite.

"Thank you. I wanted to make your favorite."

Josh grins with a huge mouthful and sauce on his chin. I smile back, seeing my little boy.

"Josh, have you been feeling OK lately?" I ask him.

He is quiet for a minute. "Yeah," he finally answers.

"I'm happy you went to the beach today with Carrie."

"I had a great day with her," he replies, beaming.

Josh helps me clean up the dishes. I want to ask him more, but I sense he's not ready to tell me how he's feeling.

"I'm going to chill in my room," he tells me when we're finished.

"OK, thank you for helping me clean up."

I relax a little, but I still can't shake the feeling that something is troubling my son. And as his mom, I feel so inadequate because I don't know how to help him.

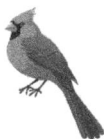

CHAPTER THREE

Prayer for Help

Help me if you can, I'm feeling down
And I do appreciate you being 'round
Help me get my feet back on the ground
Won't you please, please help me
—"Help!" The Beatles

Josh

I can't believe it's the first day of my senior year. I have walked these same halls for three years and know all of the teachers. I will be the top goalie on the varsity men's soccer team this year, and I'm dating the sweetest (and hottest) girl in school.

So why do I feel different this year?

Mom says it's because it's my last year. I notice that Mom has been asking me how I've been lately, to which I always respond, "Good." Again, that's not the truth.

I'm sad most of the time. I try to remember a happy memory of my freshman year. Nothing comes to mind. Just my sad thoughts.

There's the bell.

"How was your summer?" and high fives all around overrule Mr. Adam's attempts to get the class's attention. Carrie waves to me from the other side of the room. I still feel butterflies every time she's around. I know I love her, but I haven't told her how I've been feeling lately. I don't think she would like me anymore. She and my friends may think something is wrong with me, so I just keep how I'm feeling to myself.

We sit together at lunch, and she talks nonstop about our senior year. I'm half listening.

"Hey, Josh," Carrie asks playfully, "are you dreaming about the tropical island you are taking me to for spring break?"

"Ah, oh yeah, guess I was off somewhere," I say sheepishly, smiling at her.

"Well, you can make it up to me with a kiss." She leans over the table to meet me halfway. I get up, leaning toward her, and give her a quick kiss. She always knows how to make me feel better.

"See you later," she sings.

"Bye," I respond with a wink.

I realize I don't even like school anymore. I've never been a huge fan, but now I just want the year to be over.

It's tiring pretending that everything is OK. I pause at the classroom door and breathe.

After English class, my teacher Ms. Jenkins calls to me as I reach the door.

"Josh, everything OK?"

"Yes," I offer with a shrug.

She's always been very intuitive. *Can she sense that I am feeling bad?* Maybe I need to ask for help if it's this noticeable. *But who's the best person to ask? It should be my parents. Maybe Carrie.*

After a seemingly never-ending first day, I walk by myself to my car and get into my beat-up, hand-me-down midnight blue Volvo. Blasting the car stereo I put in last Christmas, I head home. A million thoughts still race through my head, drowning out the music.

Will I ever feel better? Will I ever be my old happy self again? Will Carrie still like me if she knows the truth about how I'm feeling?

I turn up the radio, but I can't escape my sad thoughts.

I start to cry, and I can't stop.

Sitting in the driveway, I don't even hear the lyrics of the songs playing in the background. After a few minutes, I use my shirtsleeve to wipe away years of tears.

God, I know I have not talked to you much, but I need you to help me. Something feels broken inside, and I don't know how to fix it. I'm so tired, and my body hurts every day. I'm so sad all the time. Why am I feeling this way? Mom prays to you all the time. She said you have helped her through many things. Please help me to feel like myself again.

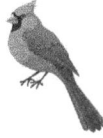

CHAPTER FOUR

A Mother's Memory

Maria

Sitting watching Josh's game, I feel sadness knowing this is his last year to play soccer in high school. Josh walks out onto the field. I feel so proud and grateful for my bright, kind, wonderful, and talented son. I watch him kick a few balls and then block several practice shots kicked by Alec on goal.

I feel tears well up in my eyes. *Get it together, Maria—is this just my worry that every time Josh goes onto the soccer field he may get hurt, or is it my wondering about how he is feeling now?*

Janet is walking toward me, and I motion to her to sit next to me.

"Hi, great to see you!" I tell her.

"You too," she replies. "Looks like I just made it."

Just then, the referees walk onto the field, and the players take their positions.

Josh blocks several goals. With his goal kick, he sends the ball soaring right to Alec. Alec maneuvers the soccer ball past several players and is in position to score. He kicks the ball and an opposing player tackles him and he falls.

"Oh, Alec!" Janet gasps.

The coaches run on to the field.

Just then, I see Josh lying on the field when he was twelve …

"Oh, Josh!" I scream. He has been hit by another player in the goalie box.

I run out to the field. Josh has been unconscious for several minutes now. All three coaches are on the field, and EMS is on its way. I'm holding back my tears; I want to be strong for my son when he wakes up. *But he isn't waking up!*

God, please help Josh wake up. Please let him be OK.

The EMS team works quickly. They check Josh's vitals and put on a neck brace. They carefully lift him and put him on the backboard. Carrying him on the backboard, they put him into the ambulance. I continue to cry as I walk toward the ambulance. They're not allowing either Aaron or me to ride to the hospital with Josh. Aaron runs to get our car so we can follow. When we get to the hospital, he drops me off at the front door. I race inside, and the front desk clerk allows me back into the emergency room area. They have transferred Josh to a hospital bed. As I walk into the room, he opens his eyes.

"Oh, Josh!" I exclaim.

"Hi, Mom, where am I?" Josh asks.

The doctor entering the room answers for me. "Hi, Josh, I'm Dr. Jones. You're at Greenville Medical Hospital. You were hit pretty hard by another player and were unconscious until you woke up just now."

"Wow, my head really does hurt." Josh exhales as he touches his head.

"We will give you something for the pain, and we will be running some tests," the doctor tells us, and then exits the room.

A nurse comes in to give Josh pain medicine to make him comfortable. Aaron walks in the room, and I explain to him that the doctor met with Josh and will be running some tests. The nurse comes back about a half an hour later to take Josh to get an MRI. Josh seems unaffected by that news, but my motherly instinct kicks in. I go over to the side of the bed to hold his hand.

"Josh, this is just a routine test so they can rule out any serious effects of the concussion," I explain.

"Mom, I'll be fine," Josh reassures me. The nurse wheels him out of the room.

But I've already done some research while waiting, and I'm less than sure. One CBS News article states that scientists already know that a concussion somehow throws crucial brain chemical reactions out of whack. However, they are not certain how long this lasts or if this imbalance could cause a chain reaction that leads to later problems, such as depression. The most obvious symptom of a concussion is a loss of consciousness that lasts from a few seconds to a half hour or more, but this doesn't always occur. Other symptoms include confusion; a persistent headache; cognitive problems; fatigue; and changes in mood, vision, or hearing. Also particularly crucial is short-term memory loss, and the longer the period of amnesia, the worse the concussion.

One thing I know is that we will be taking this very seriously. Both Josh's dad and I agree that he won't be going back to practice or playing games anytime soon.

Just then, the doctor is back with the results of the MRI.

"Looking at the scan, I do not see any permanent damage. However, as a precaution, no physical activity for two weeks." The doctor looks over at us. "If he has a loss of consciousness, persistent dizziness, or migraines, please head to your local hospital. Do you have any questions?"

"Not at this time. Thank you, Doctor," Aaron responds.

I have more questions, but I don't want to upset Josh. I will reach out to the doctor later.

We drive the three hours home, after a very long day at the hospital.

The coach calls that night to check on Josh.

"Hi, Coach. We kept Josh awake the whole ride and for another hour after we got home. He just went to bed. Thank you. We really appreciate you checking in on him."

As soon as I hang up the phone, I head upstairs to check on my son.

He is sound asleep.

I watch him for several minutes to make sure that he's OK. It's the first time I have really felt afraid for one of my children. I head downstairs to have a glass of red wine and try to relax with a movie. Our sweet Jack Russell terrier, Buddy, keeps me company.

I must have fallen asleep because the movie is over, and it's two o'clock in the morning. Turning off the television, I head upstairs to check on Josh again before going to bed. He's snoring loudly; I smile. I quickly brush my teeth, put on my pajamas, and crawl into bed.

"Thank you, God, for protecting our son," I whisper.

I realize that seeing Alec get hit brought back the memory of when Josh was knocked unconscious.

I feel the fear I felt then engulf me. I know it's the same fear that I feel now, thinking about Josh and how he's struggling with his sadness.

I see Janet out on the field next to Alec. Josh is near Alec too.

Alec sits up, and the coaches and Josh help him to his feet. Both teams start clapping in unison to acknowledge that Alec is OK.

God, thank you that Alec isn't hurt. And thank you for the memory of when you were with Josh. Please be with him now, just as you were then.

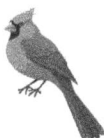

CHAPTER FIVE

Illusion of Happiness

Maria

I put on my witch's hat and black dress. I always like to get into the Halloween spirit. Lighting my new cinnamon candles, I enjoy the smell of fall filling my house. *Hocus Pocus*, the movie, is playing in the background.

AJ is already dressed as a skeleton. "Mom, I need an old pillowcase so I can go trick-or-treating with my friends," he announces, excited as a little kid.

"In the upstairs hall closet on the top-left shelf—take one of the older green ones," I reply. He happily runs upstairs in search of his candy catcher.

Audra went over to her best friend's house to help hand out candy there. Josh wants to be Frankenstein, and his dad is helping him with his makeup. He promised he would stop by to show me before going to a friend's party.

I'm opening the bags of candy to throw in a bowl for the trick-or-treaters when Josh comes barreling through the front door.

"Mom!" he yells.

"I'm in the kitchen, Josh."

"What do you think?" he asks, smiling just a bit so as to not mess up his face.

"You look fantastic!" I respond enthusiastically. He really does look great.

"I'll be right back down," he says as he runs up the stairs to his room.

Just then, the doorbell rings with the first trick-or-treaters. I pick up Buddy so he won't bark at our visitors.

"Trick or treat," say Woody and Buzz Lightyear in unison.

Josh is ready to go as I close the front door.

"Be home by 11:30 tonight," I say hopefully.

"Midnight, Mom," Josh counters.

"OK, have fun."

I want him home by midnight at the latest. I know he's a good kid, and while I've had the conversation about "don't do drugs, and don't drink and drive" with him several times, I just want to know he is safe. Josh leaves, and trick-or-treaters continue ringing the doorbell all night. My favorite is the kid who created his own robot costume out of cardboard boxes and dryer tubes all painted silver.

AJ comes home with a pillowcase full of candy that he dumps on the living room floor like he always does. He starts sorting the candy into piles by kind: Snickers, Reese's Peanut Butter Cups, Hershey's chocolate with almonds and without, Skittles, etc.

"Wow, look at all your candy!"

"You can have the Hershey's with almonds, Mom," he responds.

"Thank you, my favorite." I smile, acknowledging my youngest son's big heart.

I must have fallen asleep on the couch because Josh stumbling through the front door wakes me up. He's back before midnight, but he isn't himself.

"Hey, Mom," he manages to say, slurring his words. I can tell that Josh isn't drunk, but he has taken something.

"How was the party?" I question him.

"Fun ... going ... bed," he stammers as he trips up the stairs.

What do I do now? I call his dad. No answer. I head upstairs.

After brushing my teeth, I get in bed and just stare at the ceiling.

I know I will have to confront Josh in the morning, but I also know getting upset with him now will make matters worse.

"How do I get my point across to him?" I ask no one. Tears well up quickly.

It seems I'm crying a lot lately. I feel so unequipped to be a single mom of teenagers.

It encourages me knowing that Josh has happy moments, such as when he left for the party. I don't want to take that away from him by bringing up a tough conversation, but he needs to know the negative impact of doing drugs.

Fear creeps in, and I breathe in and out to dispel my anxiety.

I close my eyes and pray for sleep.

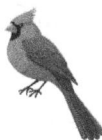

CHAPTER SIX

The Weight of Depression

There is a road, no simple highway ...
That path is for your steps alone ...
But if you fall, you fall alone ...
If I knew the way I would take you home.
—"Ripple," Grateful Dead

Josh

Lying in bed, I really don't want to get up. I keep having the same thoughts running through my mind.

How can anyone understand that I feel this way all the time now? I feel so sad, beyond any sadness that I've ever felt before. It feels like my heart has given up. And my whole body feels tired.

I sit up, then lie back down, giving into the exhaustion.

I decide to try praying to God again. "God, please take away the pain. It hurts too much!"

I'm not really sure what to believe. Does God even hear me?

The day after Halloween, Mom found seven Xanax pills—which I had taken several of the night before—in my school bag. They're so easy to get on the internet; I use my Bitcoin to purchase them from the underground drug market. I recently started taking the pills because I don't know what else to do with this overwhelming depression. The night of the party, I offered some to Alec and our buddies Zach and Mark, who we are planning to room with at Clemson University in the fall. Zach and Mark each took one, but Alec declined and told me not to take any. I did anyway, because they make me feel better. I have felt alone, and I feel accepted by my peers when I take the pills.

When Mom found them, she told me she was disappointed in me and took the pills away. I wanted to scream that I didn't want to take drugs. *They just help me feel anything but sad. I really do want help, but it feels really hopeless for me.*

With Christmas coming up in a few weeks, I don't want to make my family sad either. I used to love Christmas; I like the lights and even the silly holiday music.

Mom wants me to help decorate the tree when they get back. They really don't need my help, but Mom loves for all of us to be together.

Maybe they will come back and decorate the tree without me, I think to myself. *I really just want to go back to sleep.*

I must have drifted off because I wake up to a commotion downstairs.

I stay in bed a little while longer. I can hear my family bringing in the tree, but I'm left with my thoughts. It's hard to talk to my friends. They really don't know what to say to me. While she doesn't fully know what is going on inside my mind, Carrie wants to help. She tries to make me laugh by sending me silly cards. I pick one of her cards up off my bedside table and stare at the picture of a snowman on the front. I open the card and read the joke: *Why was the snowman rummaging in the bag of carrots? He was picking his nose.*

This makes me smile, but the happiness is always fleeting.

Nothing really helps to make the pain go away. It feels like sharp stabs of a knife constantly cutting my mind, my heart, and my body. *Maybe it would be better to make it all stop, and just end the pain. I know that would make my parents, family, and friends very sad. But I just don't see any other way.*

I force myself to get out of bed and go downstairs to help decorate the tree.

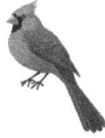

CHAPTER SEVEN
Together Yet Apart

Maria

Christmas lights twinkle through the neighborhood as I drive home, casting multicolored shadows across the dashboard. For as long as I can remember, December has been my favorite month—the traditions, the togetherness, the sense of magic in the air. This year should be no different, yet beneath my holiday enthusiasm runs an undercurrent of worry that I can't shake. Every time I think of Josh, that familiar knot forms in my stomach. Still, I force myself to focus on the joy of the season.

I do love Christmas, I think as I arrive home.

This year, I have the gifts already wrapped. AJ and Audra are excited to have a live Christmas tree. When my brother and I were kids, Mom always got us a live tree, and I have forever loved the clean pine scent they bring into our home. Living in the South now, I buy a live tree in a pot for Christmas and then plant it in January. For twelve years, I've bought everything from a magnolia tree to a holly tree and even a queen palm tree. Six of the twelve trees are still living in my front and back yards. My first "Southern" Christmas tree was a magnolia tree that is now as tall as my house.

This year we will get a cut evergreen tree since we will be moving soon; *that's an entirely different story.*

I wanted to ask Josh to go with us to pick up the tree, but he was still asleep. He spends all his time in his room, and he sleeps a lot.

I know he's depressed.

I have narrowed down the top psychiatrists near our home and scheduled an appointment for Josh in two weeks. He will not be happy about it, but he needs to talk to someone and start taking antidepressants. I will wait to tell him until after Christmas.

I smile remembering that Audra and I found AJ standing in front of a perfectly shaped Christmas tree at the nursery.

When we arrive home, Josh is still up in his room. AJ gets the tree off the car and into the tree stand. Audra puts on the lights and garlands. Now it's time to add the ornaments from years past: the beaded candy cane Audra made at six; the "baby's first Christmas" decoration from the year Curt was born; the silver reindeer I had when I was a kid; Josh's bear with the soccer ball; and of course, the Christmas pickle, which is AJ's favorite.

Josh emerges sleepily from his room. He helps put on some of the ornaments, and I smile as he does. I play Christmas music and make them all hot chocolate even though it is seventy degrees outside.

I miss the snow at Christmastime. Growing up in Pennsylvania, I woke up to many white Christmases. During Christmas in Charleston, I had to get used to what was often spring weather.

While I'm happy that Josh joined us, I hate that he is so sad. I want Christmas to be special for all of my kids. *I am grateful that we are making new memories together.*

I fall asleep remembering these new memories ... Am I dreaming? Where am I ?

I have looked at my watch fifty times today. Work is dragging, and I'm ready to leave. It's only three o'clock in the afternoon, but I start gathering my things to go home. My intuition is nudging me to pack up to leave.

My cell phone starts ringing. It's Aaron, and he's talking way too fast.

"Slow down, I can't understand you," I manage to say.

"Josh is not at school. Did you pick him up?" Aaron yells into the phone.

"No, I'm still at work. Why isn't he at school?"

Aaron has picked Josh up from middle school for the past two and a half years.

"I'm in the school office, and they're asking his teachers if he was here today," Aaron continues. "Then they're going to check the school videotape. Can you go home to see if he's there?"

"Yes," is all I can get out. I quickly email my boss and grab my things.

I'm crossing the bridge from downtown Charleston to Mount Pleasant when my cell phone starts ringing again.

"Is this Mrs. Martin?" the man on the line asks me.

"Ah, yes," I respond.

"This is Officer Johnson. Are you or someone else at home?" he continues.

"I'm driving home. Now." My voice trembles.

"I will meet you there, ma'am."

"Yes." I can barely speak as fear grips me.

I call Curt to explain what's happening. I ask him to meet AJ at his bus stop and take him to a neighbor's house. When I pull up to my house, the officer's patrol car is parked out front.

"Good afternoon, ma'am," he announces.

"Hi," I whisper.

He follows me to the front porch.

"I want to go through the house with you to look for your son and discuss where else he might have gone, if he's not home."

"Can you give me a minute to talk to my daughter?" I ask. "She didn't answer her phone when I called in my car."

The officer agrees that I can go in. I open the door and head upstairs to my daughter's room.

"Hi, Audra, can you come out?"

"Sure, Mom. What's up?" Audra asks. "Why are you crying?"

I share with her all I know about Josh leaving school. She hugs me, holding back her own tears. I'm still crying as we walk downstairs together. The officer explains he's going to search the house and then ask me some questions.

After the officer searches every room and outside the house, he comes back into the kitchen. "I would like to compile a list of all Josh's friends and their parents' names and contact numbers."

I start saying out loud the names of every friend I can think of, and Audra helps me make a list. The officer calls his partner and gives the first family's name and number. They call or visit each home in search of Josh.

I excuse myself and go upstairs. I lie on my bathroom floor and just cry.

Where could Josh be? Why did he leave school?

"Mom, are you in there?" Audra yells from the other side of the bathroom door.

"Yes," I answer.

Audra comes in and hugs me again. I have to be strong for my children, but my daughter is comforting me.

"Thank you for checking on me. Give me a few more minutes, and I will be down."

I get up and look in the mirror at my tear-stained face.

"God, please help!" I close my eyes as another tear rolls down my cheek.

I muster the courage to go back downstairs.

It's now seven o'clock in the evening, four hours after Josh would normally be leaving school.

Curt and AJ are back home. Curt put an announcement on Facebook.

"Mom, there are a lot of people looking for Josh," he shares to cheer me up.

Friends are sending text messages with words of encouragement too. But I feel numb. *The concussion a few months ago could be affecting him now. He has been a little withdrawn, now that I think about it.* Fear grips me, and I have to tell myself to keep breathing.

God, please be with Josh, and bring him home. "And whatever you ask in prayer, you will receive, if you have faith." I recall the verse in the book of Matthew.

Just then, Curt yells, "One of the moms said her daughter thinks she saw Josh at the soccer fields."

"Who?" I don't want to get my hopes up, but I hope they are right.

Aaron was asked to stay at the school with another officer while they searched for Josh. I call him to tell him what Curt read on Facebook.

"Oh, that's great news. Josh's coach is here at the school with me. I will have him go over to the fields now!"

I exhale all the fear and stress from my body. I smile at Curt and Audra to let them know that I'm staying positive. Ten excruciating minutes go by, and then the phone rings.

"Coach found him!" Aaron exclaims. "The police have to bring him to the school, and I will bring him home."

The forty-five minutes it takes to bring Josh home feel like a lifetime. He's lying in the back seat of his dad's car. Just seeing my son lying there motionless is so painful. I open the back passenger door, and Josh sits up. I get into the back seat next to him. We both sit in silence. I put my arms around him and just hug him. I can't let go.

He starts to cry. We both cry together. Josh doesn't let go either.

I wake up suddenly and sit up in bed. I'm disoriented, and I try focus on a photograph on my dresser of the kids at Curt's graduation.

My heart pounds against my ribs as I try to steady my breathing. These nightmares have been more frequent lately—vivid replays of the days when Josh was hurt or went missing.

I reach for the glass of water beside my bed, my hand trembling slightly. The Christmas tree lights downstairs cast a faint glow that creeps under my bedroom door. Earlier, watching Josh help decorate had given me hope—a small glimpse of the son I've been missing. But the dream reminds me how fragile that hope really is.

I slide out of bed, walk to the dresser, and pick up the graduation photo. All four of my children smiling back at me, Josh's arm thrown casually around Curt's shoulder. That was before. Before the sadness took hold of him. Before I started waking up in cold sweats, terrified of what might happen.

"Just a memory," I whisper to myself, tracing Josh's face in the photograph.

I place the photo back on the dresser and return to bed, knowing sleep will be impossible for the rest of the night. Tomorrow, I'll call that psychiatrist and move Josh's appointment up. Christmas spirit can only carry us so far—my son needs more than holiday magic to heal what's broken inside him.

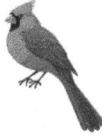

CHAPTER EIGHT

A Gift of Love

Josh

It's Christmas morning, and I'm up early, just like when I was a little kid. I smell cinnamon rolls—my favorite. Mom makes them every Christmas morning. As I walk down the stairs, I hear Mom singing along with the Christmas music: "Santa Baby." I peek around the corner into the study and see presents overflowing from under the Christmas tree.

Mom is amazing. She's up so early to put all the presents under the tree, and she makes Christmas so special for us.

"AJ, is that you?" Mom asks.

"It's me," I answer.

"Oh, Josh, Merry Christmas!"

When I walk into the kitchen, Mom greets me with a big smile. I smile back and see breakfast fresh out of the oven.

"You get the first cinnamon roll," she announces, as if I had won the lottery.

"Thanks, Mom." They are delicious.

Just then, Audra and AJ come barreling down the stairs.

"Merry Christmas," Mom sings.

"Merry Christmas! Let's open our presents!" AJ calls out as he goes to the study to check out his loot.

Mom turns up the Christmas music as Audra, AJ, and I start opening our gifts. I let myself be with my family, and I'm happy we're opening presents together.

I quickly discover that Mom got me a new phone.

"Thank you, Mom." I get up to hug her. I hold on a little longer.

She hugs me back. "You're welcome, Josh."

We all laugh as AJ puts on the silly Christmas hat that Nana sent.

After all the gifts have been opened, I help Mom pick up the wrapping paper and bows.

"Josh, remind Carrie that Christmas dinner is at four o'clock."

"I will. Thanks for inviting her."

I head upstairs to take a nap. I set my alarm to give me enough time to shower and get ready before Carrie arrives.

The alarm wakes me up. I hurry to shower and shave.

I put on khakis and a green button-down shirt. When I head downstairs, Mom is still in the kitchen.

"Can I help with anything?" I ask.

"Yes, can you carve the ham and set the table?"

"Sure," I respond as I look for the carving knife. I carve the ham and place it on the Christmas platter.

As I finish setting the table and lighting the candles for Mom, the doorbell rings.

"I'll get it!" I yell to Mom.

When I open the door, Carrie is smiling, holding a bag of gifts.

"Hi! Merry Christmas!" she greets me.

"You too," I reply. "Let me help you." I take the bag and follow her into the kitchen.

"Merry Christmas, Mrs. Martin," Carrie pronounces cheerfully.

"Merry Christmas, Carrie. I'm so glad you can join us for dinner. Thank you for the presents." Mom smiles, accepting the gifts.

"Thanks for having me."

"AJ and Audra, dinner is ready," Mom calls out.

After everyone is sat at the table, Mom says the blessing, and we start passing the food.

"Carrie, Josh said you were accepted to Wofford College. Congratulations!" Audra says to Carrie.

"Thank you! I'm so excited," Carrie exclaims.

"Hopefully Josh will get a response from Clemson University soon," Mom interjects.

I shrug nonchalantly, but in my heart I really hope she's right.

Mom tells the story of when we lost power at Christmas, and all we had to eat was the pre-cooked ham and pecan pie that she had made the night before. I smile as I think about playing Uno with my brothers, sister, and Mom and Dad by candlelight that Christmas.

After dinner, Carrie and I decide to watch *How the Grinch Stole Christmas* with everyone. Carrie has her head on my shoulder. My siblings are laughing. Mom looks so happy that we're all together. I love my family and being with them.

I can get through this hard time. *Thank you, God, for showing me how loved I am.*

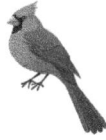

CHAPTER NINE

Unimaginable Fear

Maria

Very early in the morning, a loud noise wakes me up. *Did something fall from the roof? Or did a tree hit the house?*

I jump out of bed and quickly open my bedroom door. There is a white note propped against the spindle and a rope tied to the banister overlooking the first floor. I lean over and catch a glimpse of my second son. He's hanging from the rope.

My heart stops. I scream, or so I think. I can barely breathe.

"HELP! OH GOD, NO! HELP!" I yell out, rushing downstairs to help Josh.

I grab one of the tall kitchen chairs to put under his feet. My hands are shaking as I carry the chair and race toward my son. Josh falls to the ground. With superhuman strength, he must have used one hand to hold on to the banister and, with the other hand, loosened the rope from his neck.

I hug him as he collapses, and I can't let go. Josh doesn't seem to be present; he feels limp in my arms. I look into his eyes. He's somewhere else, very far away. Hot tears are streaming down my face. "NO! NO! NO! Stay with me, Josh!" I sob loudly.

My oldest son, Curt, comes running out of his downstairs bedroom. Seeing the look on his face, I start crying harder.

"Call your dad!" I shout to him.

Curt runs to get the phone as I rock my son back and forth in my arms.

Aaron rushes over, and we drive Josh to the emergency room. I don't know why we didn't call 911. I cannot stop crying all the way to the hospital. I'm in a cold sweat and very disoriented after the adrenaline rush. I can barely see through my tears.

We race into the emergency room, and they admit Josh.

We sit next to Josh's bed in the ER. He has been in and out of sleep all day.

I watch Josh sleep, but I keep seeing how lifeless his face was when I held him earlier.

"We could have lost him," I whisper to his dad.

Aaron just nods. He's in shock too.

I start crying again. I feel anxiety grip me and sobs erupt, and I try to gasp for air.

Breathe, Maria. Breathe.

Finally, the doctor walks into the room. He orders an MRI to rule out any injury to Josh's neck or spine. Not a single doctor could explain how Josh was able to pull himself up and get the noose from around his neck. I had seen my son hanging by his neck and with his hands at his side before I raced down the stairs. The rope was still tied to the banister.

I must have dozed off. Did I yell out? I've woken Josh up. I'm having nightmares already.

I really need to take a walk and have a moment to myself, but I can't leave my son's side.

Josh does not speak to us. He sleeps or stares off into space. He only nods or shakes his head in response to the doctor's and nurse's questions. The doctor tells us that Josh will be admitted to the Medical University of South Carolina's adolescent psychiatric unit. He's only seventeen years old.

"We love you and want to help you get better," I exclaim as I wrap my arms around him.

Josh doesn't hug me back. I see a tear roll down his cheek.

It takes every ounce of courage I have to leave his hospital room. I get a cup of coffee from the cafeteria. I stare at the white swirls from the cream in my cup, and I think of clouds at the beach.

I must be going crazy. I'm here at the hospital with Josh. The caffeine fights my exhaustion.

When I get back to the hospital room, Josh is asleep.

The nurse reassures me that she will call me if anything changes and encourages me to go home and get some sleep. I cry all the way home.

I take melatonin and rub lavender-infused lotion all over my arms, face, and neck. I lay down on top of my covers, and sleep envelops me.

The next morning, I wake up and wonder how it's possible that I slept so soundly. I get up and quickly shower and drive back the hospital. As I'm crossing the Arthur Ravenel Jr. Bridge into Charleston, it's foggy, and I see sun peeking through the clouds. All of a sudden, a full rainbow stretches over the bridge in a perfect arc. I want to see this as a sign of hope that Josh will be all right, but my mind keeps returning to seeing my son hanging.

I shudder, and my hands shake so hard. I hold the steering wheel tight and try to focus on driving. *Maria, focus on the road.*

When I get to Josh's room, Aaron is already there.

"Hi. Morning," Aaron greets me.

"Hi, where is Josh?" I question, looking back at the door.

"He just went to the bathroom."

"Has he said anything this morning?" I ask.

"He still won't talk." Aaron looks extremely sad.

Just then, Josh walks in the room. "Hi, Mom."

"Hi, Josh, good morning." I walk over to give him a hug. He hugs me back.

"Hey, Dad," Josh says, acknowledging Aaron. Josh goes over his dad, and they hug.

Aaron starts crying, and tears wet my face again too.

I am worried that Josh is not himself. *He is acting like nothing happened. I wonder how he is really feeling.*

The nurse comes back with the doctor. Josh looks away and stays quiet the whole time the doctor is speaking.

The doctor looks at me and Aaron. He seems really concerned. He rubs his forehead over and over again.

"Josh's MRI looks good, and I don't see any permanent damage. However, as discussed earlier, a minimum of one week in the psychiatric unit is necessary while he starts antidepressants and therapy."

After moving Josh to the unit, the psychiatrist says that he could come home after a week. I plan to visit him every day. However, I really don't know if he will be ready to come home in a week.

Josh has been given a new chance to live. As his mom, I want that for him more than anything.

The psychiatrist gives Josh Prozac to help with his depression. Because we discovered that he had taken a large amount of Xanax the morning I found him, Aaron and I take the opportunity to talk to him again about not self-medicating with illegal drugs as a way to feel better.

Josh just nods, listening to us.

Will he continue to self-medicate? Will he try to take his life again? God, please help my son!

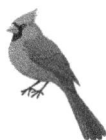

CHAPTER TEN

Facing Reality

I think I'm falling ...
It seems I found the road to nowhere ...
But I'm down to one last breath ...
Hold me now
I'm six feet from the edge and I'm thinking
Maybe six feet ain't so far down.
—"One Last Breath," Creed

Josh

I feel my body—it's very heavy. I open my eyes and see Mom and Dad sitting next to me.

Wait, where am I? I realize I'm in a hospital bed.

I'm so tired, and my neck really hurts. *Oh, I remember ... Oh no—I'm still here!*

How did I have the strength to pull myself up and loosen the noose?

How long have Mom and Dad been here? Even while feeling their unwavering love, the awful sadness is still with me.

I'm alive, but I don't want to be in this hospital bed with these itchy sheets antagonizing my skin. That's how life feels. *I don't want to be alive. Now what do I do?*

"I love you," Mom whispers as I drift off to sleep.

When I wake up again, I hear my parents asking the doctor questions.

One question particularly stands out. "When will a bed be ready so they can move him to the unit?"

Where? What? The questions are on my lips, but I can't ask them.

I drift in and out of sleep. When I finally open my eyes again, I see Mom crying. I want to tell her that everything will be OK.

But I can't do that. I don't want to talk or be awake. I don't want to be here at all.

The nurse asks me if I want something to eat. I shake my head no and close my eyes.

I wake again to Mom's scream. She has her head in her hands.

Dad tells me that they are going to move me to the adolescent psychiatric unit the next day.

What? Do they think I am crazy? I am not crazy!

Dad sees my panic and tries to assure me that they can help me there by finding the right medication for my depression.

I know and understand that I am depressed, so to be honest, I feel some relief.

I sleep off and on all night. I realize that Mom and Dad have left during the night.

The next morning, the nurse and the doctor come back to let us know that a room is ready.

I really don't want to go to the crazy floor, I think to myself but can't voice out loud. The room they take me to turns out to be even more depressing than I could imagine.

Seriously, they are the ones who are crazy. How can this help me? I want to scream, but I mumble under my breath instead.

A new nurse shows me to my room and introduces me to my roommate.

"Hi, I'm Tom."

"Hey, I'm Josh." This really sucks.

Mom and Dad say goodbye, telling that they will come to visit. I am told I will be in here no more than a week. I wave them both off, but I really don't want either one of them to go. After they leave, I go to my room and lie down. I sleep on and off all day. They force me out for dinner, followed by group therapy.

I'm so unhappy here. To make matters worse, I'm up all night because Tom snores and talks in his sleep.

Mom comes to visit me this morning and hugs me hard.

I can't hold back the tears anymore.

"Oh, Josh, I love you. We will do anything to help you get better!" Mom exclaims.

I hug her tight as I cry. "I know, Mom. I love you too," I whisper. "I'm sorry."

I can't wait to get out of this extremely depressing place. The walls are beige, and there are no pictures. And there are not enough windows. *It's definitely a prison.*

Mom or Dad come to see me every day. A week later, Dad comes to pick me up and takes me to Mom's house. It's the house I have lived in since I was five years old, and it holds too many memories.

I think about all the times I've been sad and felt so alone and about the times my parents argued. *I don't like living here without them both together.*

I sleep all day and some of the night. Mom sits with me and talks to me, but I really just want to be alone. Mom and Dad continue to make me take antidepressants and see a therapist weekly. Neither is helping. I play along, but I feel the same.

Carrie calls me when I get home from the hospital to tell me she is so thankful I'm alive. She says she loves me and assures me that I can talk to her about anything. I know she means well, but I don't want to see her yet.

What can I say? She won't understand how I feel. She is the happiest person I know.

Weeks go by, and every day is the same.

It's Easter morning, and Mom, Audra, and AJ have gone to church. I head into the backyard and open the cooler where I keep the bong I made. Getting high helps me sleep and feel better. Smoking pot gives me some relief from the sadness. It also helps me deal with stress: like from studying for exams and writing papers and telling Carrie that I always want to be with her but really don't want to go to prom.

Unfortunately, Mom comes home sooner than I thought she would. "Josh, what are you doing? How could you do that when you promised you wouldn't? Josh, I love you, and you're always welcome in my home. But you cannot smoke weed and stay here."

I say nothing in response and go to my room to get away.

Basically, she is kicking me out. I will just move in with Dad. Dad travels a lot, so that's why I have been staying with Mom. Dad's a little more understanding, but he really doesn't like me smoking pot either.

I don't know what the big deal is. It's not like I'm taking hard drugs or drinking alcohol excessively, and marijuana is legal in many states. I start packing up my clothes and things.

While I'm focused on getting out of Mom's house, Carrie is blowing up my phone. She's upset with me that I don't want to go to prom. I've always thought that prom is a waste of time and money, no matter what state of mind I'm in. *Besides, why would she want to go with me now?*

I'm not playing on my high school soccer team this spring, even though it's my senior year. It's physically and mentally too hard for me. I'm still refereeing the younger kids, which brings in good money and allows me to exercise.

I hear Mom on the phone, her voice getting louder at the end of every sentence. I know she is talking to Dad about me.

I crawl back into bed and pull the covers over my head. Sleep is my only friend.

Guess not, as listening to Mom makes it hard to sleep.

"How can we help him get better if he is just going to take illegal drugs?" I hear Mom exclaim to Dad. He just wants me to feel better, so he will tell her it's "just pot." Then she will argue that I'm too young.

I pick up my cell phone to call Carrie. I know she will tell me the same thing as Mom, but I want to hear her voice.

"Mom is kicking me out," I tell her. "She doesn't want me smoking pot."

Carrie gives me an earful since she has told me before that she doesn't like me smoking either.

I will focus on the fact that graduation is in six weeks. I have good grades, and I've been accepted to Clemson University. I just have to get through graduation, and then it's summer.

I'm ready for a change. But will college make me happier?

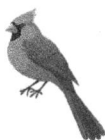

CHAPTER ELEVEN

A Mother's Love

You make my lifetime big and bright
You are my child
You came like the winds of March
With all the love in your eyes
You are my child
You came like the morning lights
With all your love, in your eyes
You are my child
—"Winds of March," Journey

Maria

God, please help Josh. He's very depressed; I feel like he's right back where he started. I pray silently as I watch the waves roll again and again onto the shore.

This is my favorite spot; here, I can breathe. I love the sacredness—I feel connected to nature, to God. I smell the salty air and see the sandpipers run to the edge of the water, darting back as the tide comes in. I listen to the sound of the waves, the rhythm calming me.

It's my favorite time of day, as the world awakens with deep orange, pink, and soft yellow kissing the sapphire blue water.

"Josh, I love you," I whisper to the sea. Thoughts of seeing Josh that awful morning cross my mind. It's been several months, and he still struggles with his sadness.

Then I remember the day Josh was born. *Twenty-four hours of labor, but so worth every minute.* He was a beautiful baby. And he was a strong baby—he lifted his head his first day of life. Josh had a head full of shiny, curly black hair that made him look older than a newborn. He had to go into the NICU—even though he was almost *ten pounds*—because he was having trouble breathing. I remember praying for him then, for his lungs to clear any fluid and for him to breathe easier.

I remember fear trying to take away my joy that day, but God answered my prayer.

Please, God, answer my prayer now. Heal Josh's mind of all sad and depressive feelings, and fill his mind with joyful thoughts. Fill his heart with your love too. I know you will always love and be there for him.

I look out at the ocean. God's love is just as deep and expansive for me, for Josh, and for Curt, Audra, and AJ.

"Curt," I whisper to the sea. My firstborn son is a young adult already. It seems like just yesterday he was playing Little League.

"Audra," I whisper again. My only daughter. She is so intelligent and kind.

Then I whisper, "AJ." I still call him my baby, even though he's an eighth grader now.

I know that I'm so blessed. My children all are gifts from God. My heart is full of love for each of them. Every hurt or heartache that my children feel, I feel too.

"How could Josh feel so lost that he would want to take his life?" I yell at the sea.

I yell at God. "God, why? How do I help my son?"

I want Josh to realize how loved he is and how important his life is to us and to God.

Then I feel guilty that I want to just enjoy my life and not have such fear and worry all the time.

The ocean breeze and the waves continue to calm me.

My peace I give to you. God's peace washes over me as I remember this scripture.

The tide is starting to come in, and the only way back from the secluded stretch of beach is to climb over the rocks. I start to navigate my journey back, but wet rocks and flip-flops don't work well together.

"Ow!" I scream. My leg slips between the rocks. Blood mixes with the salt water.

I am stuck. I strain to pull my leg free.

Just as I try again, I hear a deep voice. "Can I help?"

I attempt to turn to see who is there. "Yes," I yell as tears start to fall.

What is wrong with me? Maria, just breathe.

"Hold still." The voice is closer now. "Lean back, I've got you."

I relax and do what he asks. I feel his strong arms support me.

"I'm Grant," he says as if a friend is introducing us at a party.

"Maria," I offer in response.

"Can you move your foot out now?" he asks me with real concern.

"It's still stuck." I feel fear and frustration creep in.

"OK, I'm going to get on the rock next to you." He keeps one arm behind my back and moves to sit next to me.

Our eyes meet. He holds my gaze. His bright green eyes are gorgeous.

"Love your eyes. Green like mine," he says with ease.

Did he hear my thoughts? "Uh, thank you." *What—he likes my eyes too?*

Grant moves forward on the rock he's sitting on, and using his free arm, he gently touches my knee. I feel electricity from his hand.

"I'm going to move my hand down to your ankle and lift the rock with my other hand."

When his hand reaches my ankle, he turns to look at me.

Maria, get it together. This man is helping to free your foot.

I simply nod.

"One, two, three." He lifts the rock just enough and guides my foot free.

My hero! I look at him. "Thank you," I whisper.

"You're welcome, but let's see where the blood is coming from."

I was so enchanted with his heroism that I missed the blood now pouring from my foot.

Grant whisks his shirt off and ties it tightly around my foot to stop the bleeding.

"Once the bleeding stops, I will take a closer look. Do you feel OK?" he asks me.

"Just a little dizzy," I say. I try to stand up, and I stumble.

"Whoa! Maybe you should sit back down."

"Oh, yes," I say as I half-sit and half-fall back onto him.

"All right, let's see how bad it is." He gently removes his shirt from my ankle. "May need a stitch or two."

"Ah," is all I can get out.

"Do you think you can walk on it?" Grant questions me.

"I can try." I lift myself off the rock and find that I am able to put weight on the injured foot.

We head back to my car.

"Let's go in my Jeep," Grant offers.

"Thank you, but ..."

He smiles at me, and I smile back. Butterflies fill my stomach. *Maria, he is simply helping because you are injured.*

I nod and climb into Grant's car. We drive to the closest urgent care.

I appreciate the silence, as my mind needs a chance to catch up. My dark hair is blowing in the wind coming in through the window.

The only sounds are the hum of the car and the wind, although I'm sure he can hear my heart beating.

I'm wrapped in my favorite white silk robe with hot rollers in my hair.

When was the last time I put hot rollers in my hair? My wedding? No, I didn't do my hair then. Focus, Maria.

I smile, thinking about my date with Grant. He called to ask me out a few days after we met at the beach. We're going to one of my favorite restaurants in Charleston: Halls Chophouse. My LBD—little black dress—is already pressed. I put on nice black lingerie, my dress, and my jewelry.

"Wow, Mom. You look great," my daughter says encouragingly.

We had a long talk last night about how she felt about me going on my first date since the divorce. I know the divorce hasn't been easy on her or the boys. Audra has been open about feeling sad that her dad and I are not still married. However, she understands that sometimes parents can't stay together. I know that she loves both her dad and me, and I will continue to have open conversations with her and my sons.

"Thank you, sweetheart," I respond. I gather my purse and shoes, and we head downstairs together. "And thank you for watching your little brother tonight."

"No problem, Mom. Have fun!"

I smile and head out the front door to my car. I blast the radio and sing along to Bon Jovi's "Livin' on a Prayer" as I drive across the bridge to Charleston. I valet park and walk into the restaurant. The hostess lets me know that my date is already here.

My date. That makes me smile.

She leads me to the table. Grant stands to greet me, and I manage to say "Hi."

"You look beautiful," he says, smiling at me as he pulls out my chair.

I feel my knees go weak. "Thank you." I know I'm blushing.

He looks even more handsome than I remember. Feeling very nervous, I focus on the candlelight flickering on our table.

"How have you been?" he asks me with sweet sincerity.

"I've been good," I say, wondering if he can see through me. "And you?"

"Really good, although work has been crazy," Grant responds.

"May I ask what you do?" I look at him as I ask.

"I'm a director of an international water company."

"Wow, that sounds very interesting." I'm very impressed.

"It's a great company, and bringing water to families in towns and villages around the world is very rewarding." Grant continues to share about his work.

Our waiter comes by to get our order. Grant orders a bottle of red wine, and we give the waiter our dinner selections—we both order the filet mignon. Our conversation continues, and I learn that Grant has always lived in Charleston. The waiter brings out our meals: steak, green beans, and mashed potatoes, served in martini glasses. The red wine complements the steak perfectly. We even share a decadent chocolate cake for dessert. I could talk to Grant all night. He's genuinely interested in getting to know me and my children.

"How many kids do you have, Grant?" I question, hoping to learn about him too.

"I have a teenage daughter and a son. It's been challenging at times, raising them as a single dad."

"I completely understand. Teenagers can be difficult; the up-and-down mood swings definitely challenge my sanity."

We both laugh. I know the first date is too soon to talk about Josh's situation. However, I do allude to the fact that Josh recently moved out to live with his dad.

I excuse myself to go to the ladies' room.

I feel sadness wash over me as I think about how Josh is struggling. I allow the sadness, and I will allow the joy I feel at being on this date with Grant.

My favorite part of the evening is after dinner.

Grant suggests a stroll around Marion Square. The sweet scent of night-blooming jasmine fills the air. Spring is my favorite time of the year, coming with the promise of new beginnings. We walk through the park hand in hand. In front of a gigantic magnolia tree, Grant stops and turns toward me.

"Thank you for such a wonderful evening, Maria." He leans in and kisses me so tenderly.

I feel like I am floating.

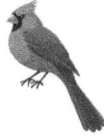

CHAPTER TWELVE

Milestones and Memories

Josh

I'm so excited to graduate today! I want this natural high more often.

Grandpa, Nana, and Aunt Rachel come into town for my graduation. So does Mom's mom—we call her "Mom-mom." They are
meeting us at the coliseum. Dad and I get into his Volkswagen to
head to my commencement.

I look over, and Dad is smiling.

"I am so proud of you."

"Thank you, Dad!"

We park, and I grab my cap and gown out of the back seat. Dad
gives me a big hug.

I walk toward the entrance of the coliseum. It will be a long
graduation. There are over a thousand kids in my class: Class of 2016.

As we process in, I feel so happy that I'm graduating. I'm excited
and nervous as I wait for the principal to call my name.

Finally, my name is called. I hear my family yell. I can't help
smiling as I head to the stage.

Mr. Thompson, my favorite engineering teacher, reaches to shake my hand. "I'm very proud of you, Josh." I know my parents and my grandparents are proud of me, but it's great to hear my teacher say he's proud of me too.

Carrie waves and smiles as I pass her row.

I smile and blow her a kiss. *My heart feels full.*

After graduation, Alec is the first person I see.

"Hey, Josh, congratulations!" He reaches to shake my hand.

"You too!" I shake his hand. "Can we get together this summer?"

"Definitely, Josh, it will be great to hang out. Enjoy your day with your family." Alec sees his family and heads toward them.

I find my family gathered in a circle outside. Everyone congratulates me.

Mom hugs me first. She wants pictures of me with everyone after my graduation. "So, let's all meet up at the park by the bridge," she announces.

I drive with Dad to Waterfront Park. It's fun taking pictures with my family. One of my favorite pictures is three generations: Grandpa, Dad, and me.

I have a brief moment of sadness remembering the day I walked out of school in eighth grade and scared my parents. I had walked all the way to this park and paced back and forth on the dock. I even walked up onto the Ravenel Bridge.

After the concussion, I've had several moments of sadness. It's gotten worse over the years, with this year being the worst. *Why do I always have sad thoughts?*

"Enough negative thoughts," I whisper to myself.

It's just a memory, and I want to be present with my family.

Mom has reserved a table at my favorite Italian restaurant for dinner. It's really nice sitting around the table with all my family. They are telling stories about me.

"I remember when Josh would sleep with his soccer ball," Dad exuberantly shares.

"And I remember when Josh was the first to reach the top of the rock wall at his tenth birthday party," Curt adds to the conversation. He looks over at me and smiles.

I feel self-conscious, but I enjoy hearing the many stories about me.

"One of my favorite memories is of Josh at the lake in Massachusetts. When the tube flipped, he started to panic, but when he realized he could just stand up, he started laughing," Aunt Rachel recalls.

After dinner, I go to the bathroom. Coming out, I almost knock Carrie over. She's there with her family too.

"Hi, Josh. Congratulations," she sings in her sweet voice. She hugs me hard.

"Congratulations to you too." I hug her back.

"Can you believe we are high school graduates?" Carrie asks.

"I know, it's pretty cool." I smile at her.

She grabs my hand, and then she kisses me on the cheek. "See you later, Josh."

"Bye, Carrie." *I wish I had the confidence to tell her that I really do love her.*

I turn and head back to the table. My family continues telling stories. I close my eyes for a moment, taking in the day.

When I look up, I see Mom smiling at me.

The summer goes by way too fast. I should be packing, but I'm sitting by the pool enjoying this perfect summer day—a bright blue sky without a single cloud. I have spent a lot of my summer at the pool at Dad's apartment complex by myself. I did hang out some with Alec too. My thoughts keep going to Carrie. This summer, she has invited me over and over again to the beach or a movie. *I always have an excuse not to go, and that makes me sad.*

"I will go to the last party of the summer," I say out loud to convince myself.

I head inside to get ready. After I shower, I pick out a fun Hawaiian shirt. I love my collection of multicolored Hawaiian shirts. I like to be different from everyone else.

"Bye, Dad," I announce as I head out the door.

"Have fun, and be home by midnight," Dad calls back.

Driving across the bridge toward the ocean is always magical. As I come over the top of the bridge, I see the sunlight shimmering on the blue water. I'm going to miss this place. I'm suddenly flooded with a myriad of memories—especially of the magical beach day with Carrie.

Turning right at the stoplight, I head to the Sullivan's Island club for my senior class pool party.

Alec pulls up right next to me in the parking lot. "Hi, Josh," he greets me.

"Hey, man!"

We walk in together. There are colorful balloons and tiki torches everywhere, with beach music creating a fun vibe. There are at least two hundred kids laughing, playing games, and swimming. And girls in bikinis everywhere. I smile, really glad that I came.

"Wanna play volleyball first?" Alec asks.

"Yes, that sounds like fun!" I yell back to be heard over the crowd.

Teams are forming, so Alec and I join in with a bunch of guys we know from school.

I really enjoy the camaraderie and the competition of the game. It's great hearing the girls cheering for us as they watch from beach chairs next to the volleyball courts.

Our team wins. After shaking hands with the guys on the other team, Alec and I walk off the court in search of food. We grab hamburgers, chips, and drinks and sit in lounge chairs by the pool.

As I look up with a huge mouthful of hamburger, Carrie is walking toward us.

"Hi, Josh. Hi, Alec," she says jubilantly.

I manage a muffled "Hi" with my stuffed mouth.

Alec waves for Carrie to come over.

"Can you believe that we'll be leaving for college next week?" she asks both of us.

"Not at all!" Alec comments. "Josh and I were just sharing stories about Mr. Jones's first-grade class."

"He started each class with calisthenics," I add, smiling at the memory. "It seems like that was just yesterday."

"I didn't have Mr. Jones," Carrie continues. "Mrs. Wheeler has always been my favorite teacher from elementary school. She read us poetry every class."

"We have had great teachers, but I'm ready for college," I share with them.

"Want to go for a walk on the beach?" Carrie suddenly asks.

"Sure, let me clean up. See you in a bit, Alec." He grins at me.

As Carrie and I walk toward the beach and down to the water, I'm deep in thought.

"How have you been, Josh?" she finally asks me.

"I'm doing really well." I surprise myself when I say it.

Carrie pauses. I stop and look at her.

"I'm doing a little better. Just not fully me yet."

"I know you have been through so much." Carrie grabs my hand. "I'm here for you."

"Thank you, Carrie."

We walk further up the beach. She stops again. I automatically move closer to her. Our lips touch, and I feel the electricity between us. Kissing Carrie is fantastic. The sun is starting to set, and we hold hands watching the sky change colors.

I know she loves me, and I will always love her.

When the sky finally gets dark, we head back to the party. Alec asks us to help get firewood to start a bonfire on the beach. Roasting s'mores and looking up at the stars with Carrie beside me, I'm reminded that life is good.

I'm starting to feel a little bit like me again.

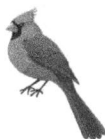

CHAPTER THIRTEEN

Time with My Son

Maria

I just received Josh's graduation pictures. Remembering Josh at his graduation brings tears to my eyes. I printed the pictures taken at Waterfront Park after his graduation. Josh looks so carefree and happy. Seeing him in one of the pictures with all of the family, against the gorgeous colors of the sunset—mauve, pink, and orange layered over the Charleston Harbor—it's like I'm there again.

Josh is coming over for a few days to pack up the things he wants to take to college. He left several of his things in his room that I have left untouched. I've asked him to go through all of his clothes and divide them into three piles: clothes for college, clothes he can take to his dad's house, and clothes for donation. I hope he decides to keep the Duke basketball jersey signed by Coach K.

I am happy that we get to spend time together. Since he's been living with his dad for several months, I've only seen him a half dozen times. I have missed him, although I'm relieved that his dad has shouldered more of the day-to-day concerns. When Josh was living with me, I would wake up often at night, worried that he couldn't sleep or that he may have taken drugs. *And the fear he might hurt himself again never goes away.*

I want the next few days with Josh to be fun and like a trip down memory lane.

I hear the front door open and close.

"Hey, Mom," Josh calls out from the foyer.

"Hi, Josh, I'm in the kitchen."

"Can we go to my favorite burger place for dinner tonight?" Josh asks first.

"Yes, that's perfect. I've been thinking about taking you to some of your favorite places over the next few days," I share happily.

"Cool. I'm going to go through most of my clothes this afternoon," Josh states.

"Let me know if I can help. We can go to dinner around six," I respond, wondering how he's been feeling. I will ask him after he settles in.

"Sounds good, Mom." Josh heads upstairs.

Driving to Josh's favorite burger place, I sense that he doesn't want to talk about his sadness.

I wish he didn't have this battle with depression.

I will enjoy the next few days with him.

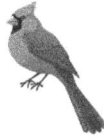

CHAPTER FOURTEEN

College-Bound

Josh

Today, I leave for Clemson. The water in the shower feels invigorating, as if each drop could give me the courage I need to go off on my own. I have to hurry; Alec will be here soon. I put on my favorite orange Clemson T-shirt and tan shorts. After getting dressed, I bring the last few bags down from my room.

"Hi, Mom. Good morning."

"Morning, Josh. Do you want some eggs?" Mom calls out from the kitchen.

"I would love some. Thanks, Mom."

I grab orange juice from the fridge and pour some into my favorite Clemson cup.

"You have everything ready to go?" Mom looks at me as she puts a plate of eggs and toast in front of me.

"It's all downstairs in the hallway, plus the bedside table and desk chair in the study."

"You ready too?" Mom asks.

"I'm ready. I know I will do well in school," I reply with confidence. "And I'm looking forward to college and having fun with my friends, too."

The doorbell rings, and I open the front door to see Alec and his dad.

"Hey, morning," I greet them both.

"Morning. Let's load up the U-Haul," Alec says, taking charge. We load my bedside table, lamp, and desk chair. Then we add all the boxes, full of my belongings.

"See you soon, man." I wave as Alec and his dad drive off.

I hold Buddy, our terrier, and tell him I will miss him. He licks my face, and I laugh.

My mom and I drive in separate cars to Clemson so I can have a car at college. I wait half an hour for her to show up on campus. I guess I do have a lead foot. We walk around campus to look at some of the buildings where I will have classes. I think Mom sees me checking out the girls we pass.

I smile at many of them, but my heart is with Carrie.

Mom takes me to lunch after we get my books.

"So, this is it," Mom finally says to me.

"Yeah, I'm really excited." I smile back at her.

"Josh, I know you will do well." Mom pauses. "And you know your dad and I are only a phone call away."

"I know. Thank you, Mom." I look down at my phone, avoiding more of her questions.

After lunch, Mom follows me to the apartment so I can check in.

I get my keys, and an upperclassman shows me my mailbox. Alec and his dad are already there. Mom's great, helping me unload my stuff and setting up my room. I can tell she is holding back tears as she stands there to say goodbye.

"Bye, sweetheart. I love you," Mom barely whispers as she hugs me tight.

"Love you too, Mom," I say loudly as I hug her back.

Mom says goodbye to Alec and his dad and to my roommates, Mark and Zach, and their parents. She waves to me and walks out the front door.

This is really it. I go to my room and plop onto my bed. I feel excited and nervous and relieved all at the same time.

I wake up when Alec jumps onto my bed.

"Time to go," he announces.

"Where are we going?"

"Our first college party," Alec states proudly.

"Oh, cool. I'll be right out."

I decide I'm going to go out with my roommates, instead of keeping to myself. Getting out of bed, I head to my bathroom. I quickly brush my hair and put on more deodorant. I change into one of my Hawaiian shirts and grab my flip-flops.

"Where's the party?" I ask.

"It's right up the hill," he says, "so we can walk."

Wow, there are hot girls everywhere, but my stomach dictates my first move. I make a beeline to the pizza and grab two slices of pepperoni. Then I get my first college beer, Bud Light, from the cooler.

There are drugs at the party too.

This is going to be a lot harder than I thought. I am offered some weed.

"Would you like some?" a friendly girl asks me.

"I'm good for now," I answer quickly.

I find Alec talking with a group of girls. I know that meeting new people is just what I need. The girls keep asking me lots of questions—I love the attention.

Thank you, Alec. I have shared with him that I want to stay away from drugs.

My first night on campus is a success.

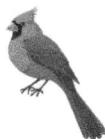

CHAPTER FIFTEEN

New Beginnings

Maria

Yesterday, I drove back from Clemson after dropping Josh off at college. I invited Grant to dinner; cooking is cathartic for me. I want my mind to be on that and on seeing Grant, and yet negative thoughts are tricky invaders. They've brought worry about Josh all day. Audra is out with her friends, and AJ is with his dad tonight.

Grant and I have gone to breakfast and lunch several times since our first dinner date. I invited him over so we can have a relaxed atmosphere in which to continue to develop our new, wonderful connection. Grant continues to surprise me with romantic gestures. He sent a bouquet of white lilies to my office last week.

I've made Cornish game hens, roasted potatoes, and asparagus. I've even made a blueberry tart for dessert. Playing my favorite French music in the background, I set the table and light the candles.

I run upstairs to put on a blue flower-patterned summer dress that accentuates my feminine curves and pull my hair up in a French twist.

I'm just pulling the food out of the oven when the doorbell rings.

"Hello," I greet Grant with a smile and kiss him on the cheek.

"Hi. Wow, you look beautiful." Grant knows how to compliment me in the sweetest way.

"Please come in." I wave him into the foyer.

Grant follows me into the kitchen. "Your house is so like you." I have decorated with bright, colorful paintings of the beach, and many feminine touches—candles in artistic candleholders; fun-shaped pillows of soft materials like silk; and curtains, whimsical and flowing.

"Thank you." I appreciate his attentiveness, wondering what specifically he noticed, but I don't ask him.

"Would you like a glass of wine? Red or white?" I gesture to the bottles on the counter.

"Yes—red, please." Grant winks at me.

I pour two glasses of red wine and start plating our dinner. "Will you help me carry the plates to the table?" I ask Grant.

"Of course. Can I help with anything else?" he questions.

"No, thank you. I will bring our wine."

"Maria, this looks wonderful."

"Thank you. Can I say a blessing?" I look up to see Grant nod in agreement.

"Dear God, bless this food to our bodies, and bless each of us and our families. Amen."

After the first bite, Grant looks up. The smile that spreads across his face expresses exactly what I'm feeling inside.

"Maria, this is absolutely delicious. Thank you for having me tonight."

"You're welcome—I'm so glad you came," I respond, smiling.

After dinner, we clear the table and wash the dishes together. Then we share the blueberry tart while continuing our conversation on my screened-in back porch. Grant reaches for my hand while he continues telling me about his grandparents, who live in Germany.

"Would you like some more wine?" I ask him.

"Let me get it," he offers, heading to the kitchen to retrieve the bottle of wine.

He pours wine for each of us and sits down beside me again.

"Cheers to new beginnings!" Grant toasts.

"Cheers," I reply, and we clink our glasses and each sip our wine.

Grant reaches out to hold my hand. It's the exact gesture I need to be open with him about Josh.

"Grant, I really want to share with you what's been going on with my second son, Josh."

I tell him everything about Josh, from his first concussion until now.

"I'm here for you." Grant squeezes my hand. "Maria, thank you for being vulnerable and for trusting me enough to tell me about Josh."

I tear up a little, and Grant puts his arm around me and kisses me.

Our evening continues with stories and sweet kisses. It's a perfect evening that I know I will always cherish.

We walk hand in hand to the front door. Turning toward me, Grant pulls me close to him. He kisses me slowly, and then more passionately. I slip easily into each kiss, wanting more.

"Would you like to go to one of the plantations with me next weekend?" Grant asks after our lips part.

"I would really enjoy that." I look into his bright green eyes.

"Can I pick you up at ten o'clock Saturday morning?" he inquires.

"Yes, that's perfect."

He kisses me slowly again. I want to stay in this moment forever.

"I had a wonderful time tonight," he whispers as our lips part again.

"I did too." I smile.

"Bye, and sweet dreams." One more kiss, and he turns to open the front door.

"You too. Good night." I watch Grant walk to his car.

He smiles again as he waves goodbye. I feel hope for the first time in a while.

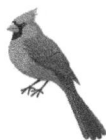

CHAPTER SIXTEEN

Call for Help

Hello darkness, my old friend ...
Because a vision softly creeping ...
And the vision that was planted in my brain
Still remains
Within the sound of silence
In restless dreams I walked alone
—"The Sound of Silence," Simon & Garfunkel

Josh

College has been fun, and I'm doing well in my classes. But I'm not sleeping again. I'm up all night, and it's a struggle to get up in the morning. Luckily, most of my classes are at midday. My one early class is Algebra II, and math is easy. The professor counts attendance, but it's only a small percentage of my grade.

My cell phone starts ringing, and I look down to see it's Carrie calling.

"Hi, Josh, how are you? How's college going?" she asks me.

"Hey, I'm good. I'm enjoying it," I tell her. "How about you?"

"I'm great. I love my school, my classes, my roommate, and my new friends."

What new friends? I want to ask.

"Come see me. It would be great to see you. And you can meet my friends." She must have known what I'm thinking.

I can feel her excitement through the phone. "Uh, that would be fun," I say clumsily.

Why am I not able to speak to her, even on the phone?

"The weekend after next is our homecoming," Carrie continues.

"Oh, it is?" I ask, wishing I could sound cool.

"Do you think you can come?" she asks.

"I'm pretty sure I can come that weekend."

She knows I hate events like that, but I really want to see her.

"Great, we can make plans later this week. I've gotta go get some homework done now. We will talk soon. Bye," she says, all in one breath.

"Bye," I say and hang up the phone. *I really do want to see her.*

I'm lost in thought, thinking about Carrie, when Alec bursts into the room.

"Let's go. Party time!" Alec shouts.

"OK, give me five, and I will be out."

My homework is done, but I'm exhausted. To be honest, I don't want to go out. I'm feeling depressed again. But I think being around people will be good for me. So, I go. I run into the pretty blond girl I see at every party. I cannot remember her name.

"Hi, you," she says, smiling her sweet smile.

"Hey," is all I can get out.

"Wanna drink?" she asks.

"Sure. I'll have a beer." I only drink two. I'm so tired.

"Wanna try this?" she asks.

"What's that?" I question.

"LSD," she responds, showing me several tablets in her hand.

"OK," I hear myself say. *Oh no, what am I doing?* I put two on my tongue.

She smiles at me. I feel the drug start to affect me.

Zach comes up to me and hands me a joint.

How many hits did I do? I am really tripping now.

I see the same girl and her friends hours later. *Or maybe it's been ten minutes.*

The girl is getting into a car, and I jump in. "Can you take me to the hospital?"

"No, get out of my car!" she screams.

I get out and stand in the street. *I feel really bad. How long have I been outside?*

Just then, an ambulance pulls up. *Did I call 911?*

Why am I restrained? I see a nurse in the room. *What day is it?*

I remember Mom was here. *Wait, what? Why was Mom here? She was sad. I saw her crying.*

How long have I been here?

Why does my head hurt so much? Is Mom coming back?

I wake up another time, and there is a new nurse, asking me questions. Do I know where I am? Do I know who I am?

Wait. What? Did I say I was someone else when I first got here?

The room is small and dark and cold—the walls are closing in on me. *I want to get out of here.*

I am lying on a very uncomfortable bed with a thin blanket. *I am freezing.*

The only other thing in the room is an annoying clock on the wall. It's the only thing I hear. *Tick, tock, tick, tock.*

Mom is here again. She is talking to the younger nurse. I can't make out what they are saying.

Did Mom say I'm getting out of here?

Oh, thank you, Mom!

Mom is gone again when I wake up. There is a tray of food on a little brown folding table next to the bed. I try to eat, but my throat is so dry. All I can do is sip the water from the tiny plastic cup. I feel like I'm going to throw up. I just dry heave instead.

Can someone please help me?

The nurse brings me my clothes and tells me to get dressed. When I sit up, I have to pee. I tell the nurse that. She tells me I have to get in the wheelchair, and then they can take me to the bathroom.

Why? I can walk. Whatever! I have to go. They bring a wheelchair.

When I'm wheeled back to the dingy, depressing room, the nurse explains that I will be going to another hospital.

What? Why?

Mom is back, and she hugs me.

Please get me out of here! I want to yell.

But I don't ask Mom why.

The next day, I'm in another bed, at another place. A doctor comes in to see how I'm doing.

"Josh. Hi, good morning. I'm Dr. Collins."

"Hi," I say back.

"Do you know why you are here?" he asks me.

"I took a lot of LSD," I answer.

"Yes, more than the legal limit."

There's a legal limit? I thought the stuff was illegal. I keep that thought to myself.

"This facility will help you detox from the drugs," the doctor explains to me. "After detoxing, you will need to continue therapy."

Wait, now I have a drug problem? I am depressed, I want to scream.

I don't see Mom the next day or the day after that.

It's complete hell.

My body shakes violently. One minute I'm hot, dripping with sweat, and then I'm freezing. I sleep terribly. My body wants to sleep all day because that's what it's used to, but they keep me awake all day.

I want to see Mom and Dad. They tell me that Dad will be here in a week to pick me up. Mom calls and says she loves me.

Then get me out of here! I want to yell into the phone, but deep inside I know that taking LSD was a huge deal. I had never taken LSD before that night.

I took it, and this is the consequence. I really just need help with my depression. Taking drugs like Xanax and marijuana is my only escape from feeling depressed all the time.

Just then, I think of Carrie. She invited me to her school. I really wanted to see her, but that isn't going to happen now. I start to cry.

God, if you are there, can you please help me be happy again?

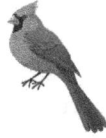

CHAPTER SEVENTEEN

Seeking Help

Maria

Thursday night, I receive the call that no parent wants to receive. The dean at Josh's college calls me to say that Josh is in the emergency room. I begin to cry. I silently pray for God to be with him. The dean goes on to explain that Josh had actually called 911 for help. He was under the influence of two types of drugs: LSD and marijuana.

Oh no! I slump down onto the kitchen floor. I force myself to breathe.

Maria, breathe in. Breathe out. Breathe in and out. I get up, continuing to breathe deeply.

I take out a glass from the cupboard and pour water from the pitcher. I swallow the first sip. And then another sip.

Gathering my thoughts, I pick up the phone, my hands trembling. I call the hospital. The front desk receptionist puts me through to a nurse in the emergency room.

"Hello, this is Maria Martin. I'm Josh Martin's mom." I frantically speak into the phone.

"Hi, Ms. Martin. Your son is here in the emergency room," the receptionist states.

"How is he?" I ask, very upset.

"They have him isolated and restrained," she says curtly.

"Restrained?" I gasp.

"It's only until he calms down," she continues.

"I will be there in the morning," I manage to respond.

Our weather is terrible, with a looming hurricane. I look out the kitchen window. It's pouring already, and the wind is blowing the limbs of my willow tree wildly.

I know I cannot drive four and a half hours tonight, being so upset and in this weather.

I wake up early. *Who am I kidding? I didn't sleep at all.*

I take a quick, cold shower to revive my courage. I grab my overnight bag and a thermos of coffee and get on the road. The phone rings.

"Hi, Aaron, good morning." I left a message for him last night.

"How is Josh?" he asks me.

"Not sure. I'm on my way to the hospital now. I will call you once I see him."

"OK, please let me know." Aaron exhales.

I hang up the phone and do my best to concentrate on driving in the rain. Several hours and many raindrop-sized tears later, I finally reach the hospital. My hands hurt from gripping the steering wheel. After finding a place to park, I walk into the hospital.

Josh is in a small room in the emergency area. A very kind nurse leads me to his room.

"Hi, Josh, it's Mom." Josh looks at me, but he doesn't know who I am. He's still very delusional from all of the drugs.

He starts rambling on and on that an alien is eating his brain and causing him so much pain. I hold his hand as he tells me this, tears streaming down my face. All I can do is be here for my son. I tell him how much I love him.

"Your dad and I will do everything we can to help you," I whisper to him.

Please, God, help my son.

I sit with him for two hours. I don't want to leave him, but he needs to rest. I stand and kiss him on his forehead, like I did when he was a little boy. Reluctantly, I walk out of the hospital, get into my car, and head to my hotel. I call Aaron on the way to let him know that Josh is going to be moved to another room and they will continue to help him safely detox from all the drugs. I reassure him that I will go back first thing in the morning. I crawl under the covers of the hotel bed and look at the clock. It's quarter to eight in the evening.

When I look at the clock again, it's six o'clock in the morning. I shower, and this time I make it scalding hot. After I get dressed, I make coffee. I drive to Josh's apartment, and Alec lets me in. We talk briefly, and I tell him where they're taking Josh. I gather his clothes, blanket, pillow, and toiletries. Then I head back to the hospital. Josh is still in the emergency area and in the same room.

WTF?

"Why is Josh still in this same confining room?" I question the nurse, trying to remain calm.

"They are transferring him to a temporary behavioral facility sooner rather than later."

"Where?" I ask.

"Springfield Behavioral Facility. They will help him continue to detox safely and start his therapy," the young nurse tells me.

I turn from her and look at my son.

"Josh, it's Mom."

"Hi." Josh looks up as he recognizes me.

The nurse begins explaining everything to him as if he's going to a new school.

Josh, with tears in his eyes, gives me a questioning look.

I try to smile through my tears. "You took too many drugs, and they can help you detox."

He looks away from me, but I catch a tear falling down his cheek.

They have to transfer Josh by ambulance. Before they come to get him, I go over and hug him. He doesn't hug me back. I follow behind as they wheel him outside.

As they put Josh in the ambulance, I shout, "I will be right behind you!"

They close the doors, and my tears fall again.

I drive the twenty minutes to the facility. Checking in at the front desk, I ask to see my son.

"Mrs. Martin, Josh has already been admitted. It's our policy that once a patient has been admitted, guests are not allowed," the receptionist says matter-of-factly.

I can't believe that they won't let me see my son.

"I will wait to talk to the doctor," I tell her.

An hour later, Dr. Collins shakes my hand briskly and tells me the facility's rules again. I will not be able to see Josh because it's part of the detox process.

"Josh is not violent, but he's having outbursts," Dr. Collins explains.

"Please let him know that I love him," I whisper. My heart sinks.

The doctor nods and walks off.

I leave Josh's clothes, blanket, pillow, and toiletries with the front desk receptionist. I have to force myself to walk out the door and leave my son there. It's the best facility in the area, but I'm not convinced that they will lovingly care for my son. I sob quietly as I walk back to my car.

I call Grant on the way back to the hotel.

"Hi, how's it going?" he asks me right away.

"Not well. Josh is in a temporary behavioral facility to help him detox," I share with Grant. "But I know he needs better care."

"I know you will find the right place for him. Go get some rest."

"I will try. Thank you for listening. Good night."

In my hotel room, I lie on my bed, staring up at the ceiling.

"God, please help Josh. I don't know what to do to help him," I whisper toward heaven.

When I wake up, it is two in the morning, it's dark, and I'm freezing. I find the light switch and go to the bathroom. I take the longest and hottest shower I have ever taken. I turn off the water and dry off. I'm thankful for the soft towels and robe. I wrap the fluffy white robe around me and tie the sash. As I wrap my hair up in a towel, I look at my tear-stained face in the mirror.

I sit back on the bed and just stare out the window, into the dark abyss of the night. All I can think about is what Josh is going through—it must be horrific.

"God, why is this happening? Why can't the doctors help Josh? Why is he so sad?" I scream, pounding my fists into the mattress as anger envelops me.

God, please ease his pain. I fall back asleep.

I wake up again at nine o'clock in the morning. I know I really needed that sleep. I quickly get ready and go in search of breakfast in the hotel lobby. I opt for black coffee and a croissant. I want to go back and see if I can visit Josh before I head home. I know that asking is futile, but I will wait to talk to the doctor again.

I tell Dr. Collins that I want my son to choose life and good health. I don't want Josh to choose drugs as a way to self-medicate his depression and pain.

The doctor looks at me like I'm crazy. "First, we have to help him detox," he says without feeling.

Wow, this is not the right place for my son. How can they be so cold and uncaring?

I honestly don't know anything about mental health or drug treatment facilities. I call Aaron as soon as I get back in the car to head home. We both agree to start researching the best place to help Josh.

The following week, Aaron drives to pick up Josh. We found a therapeutic facility in the Blue Ridge Mountains in North Carolina.

It's a wilderness addiction treatment program that will help Josh learn new skills to cope with his addiction.

Josh has a dual diagnosis of addiction and depression. Although his dad and I believe his depression is his biggest challenge, the doctors are in agreement that his addiction is the problem that needs to be treated first. The wilderness treatment center we have chosen for Josh will help him with his drug addiction and substance abuse through outdoor therapy. The wilderness creates experiences that will help Josh build confidence and become aware of himself and his patterns much quicker.

Josh told us that he stopped calling his therapist and taking his antidepressant when he started college. Since he's now eighteen, as his parents, we no longer have legal guardianship. Aaron and I went to court to seek guardianship of Josh so we could make medical and therapeutic decisions for him. The judge granted our request.

Josh is very reluctant to go to the new facility, and he asks his dad over and over again if he can come home. I know it will be heart-breaking for Aaron to leave him at the center. It would devastate me.

But Josh needs help, and every other facility is like a prison for young adults. We're afraid to put him in any state facility, fearing that they would just medicate him and not get to the root of the problem.

I'm in disbelief over how few options there are to help young adults with addiction and mental health conditions.

Aaron said he would call me after he dropped Josh off at the wilderness facility.

I am so sad for Josh. And I'm angry that finding help for him is so difficult.

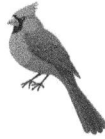

CHAPTER EIGHTEEN

Boy Scout Hell

Josh

Dad is coming to get me today. I'm so relieved to be going home. When I see Dad, I start to cry. He gives me a big hug, and I cry harder.

"I love you, Josh."

"I love you too," I whisper back.

We get my stuff and head outside. The fresh air is so wonderful after the stale air of that prison. As we drive down the long drive toward the main road, I know that I will not be heading back to college.

What am I going to do now? Can I go to another college?

"Josh, I need to tell you something. The only way they would release you from that facility is if your mom and I found the right place for you. We found a great wilderness program in the North Carolina mountains. They will teach you skills to help with addiction and depression." Dad is telling me what I'm going to be doing now.

I want to yell that I don't want to go. *Why can't I figure out how to get better on my own?* The truth is, though, I need help.

I'm silent for a while, and then I fall asleep.

Opening my eyes, I see Dad is outside the car, pumping gas. I feel groggy, but I have to use the bathroom. When Dad finishes pumping gas, we walk into the gas station together. I go to the bathroom while he gets us drinks and snacks. I wash my hands and splash water on my face.

How can my parents want to put me in another place? I just don't think that spending time in the woods is going to help me with my depression.

I walk out to find Dad waiting for me. All I want to do is run away, but instead, I get in the car.

"Dad, how much longer until we get there?" I ask without emotion.

"About an hour," he says, and it seems like he wants to say more.

"Josh, I really want to know how you have been feeling. And why are you taking drugs?"

I don't answer Dad right away. Then I find the courage to respond.

"Dad, I've been very depressed, and drugs help me feel better," I finally tell him.

Dad is silent now.

I just want to sleep.

When I wake up again, we are winding up a hill toward a lodge at the top. We park in the gravel parking lot.

"Dad, do I have to stay here?" I ask, knowing the answer.

"It will only be for a few weeks, Josh. Look at the beautiful mountains—it looks like a very nice place."

It does look nice, but I don't have a drug problem. I take drugs to escape how awful I feel all the time. I'm not convinced this place is going to help. I just want to go home.

The director meets us at the front door. "Hi, I'm Jim Wilson."

"Hi, I'm Aaron, and this is Josh." Dad shakes his hand.

"Hi, Josh, welcome." I nod back to this stranger. He shows us around the main lodge and the room where I will sleep. It's a big closet with a dresser, a bed with an ugly army green bedspread, and plaid, brown-and-white-checked curtains covering the window. We go back to Jim's office, and he tells us about the program. Dad brought me boots and warmer clothes. The director explains that they will provide an all-weather jacket, sleeping bag, tent, and all the other gear I will need.

What? I'm not a Boy Scout, I want to tell this guy.

Jim continues to explain that the first two weeks will be here at the lodge while we learn outdoor skills. Then we will set out, as a group, to the campsite.

Dad looks at me, but I don't want to make eye contact. I stare at the wooden floor, hoping Dad will change his mind.

"OK, so we are all set with the paperwork," the director says, looking at Dad before turning to me. "Josh, you ready?" he asks.

No! I want to scream. I just nod again.

I know I made the wrong choice by taking LSD. But how can treatment in the wilderness help me? Maybe I can give it a try.

Dad and I walk out onto the front porch. I stare at the Blue Ridge Mountains stacked up against the sky; they do look blue and purple.

"Josh, you're going to learn how to build a fire, cook your own meals, set up a tent, and pack everything up before hiking to a new location and setting up camp again. This program will challenge you to think and care for yourself." Dad tries to be upbeat. But I see him nervously look away.

"Josh, I love you so much. You will learn a lot here and be home before you know it." Dad is trying to convince himself with each word. He hugs me and says goodbye.

Wait! What on earth just happened? Dad's left me at some wilderness camp to cure me of an addiction problem that I don't have. Well, maybe I do have an addiction problem, but my depression is worse.

Why am I here? Learning to start a fire and tying knots can't possibly help me.

Curt was a Boy Scout, and that's fine for him. When I was younger, I told Mom that I would never join. So here I am, learning skills that I don't need.

Most of the kids here have anger issues on top of their addictions. One guy yells at the counselors all the time. I avoid him and everyone else. The counselors tell me that I have to participate, but I don't want to do anything they're asking me to do. Next week, they're going to send us out to fend for ourselves with our gear and newly learned skills.

Mom calls and says that she's found a better place for me in Tennessee.

"Mom, I just want to come home." I try to hold back my anger.

"I understand, Josh, but you need help with your depression and addiction. I'm sorry that they can't help where you are now. The people at the new place have reassured me that they can help with your depression."

"I really don't want to go, and I hate you for making me do any of this." I hang up.

I feel sick to my stomach. *Why can't they help me here now?* I'm mentally and physically exhausted and very depressed.

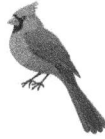

CHAPTER NINETEEN

Searching for Sanctuary

Maria

Within a week, we receive a call from the director to say that their program is not the right solution for Josh. With his suicide attempt earlier this year and the fact that addiction is not his only issue, they will not be able to help our son.

Are you kidding me? Really, they knew his situation, and the previous doctor had said that his addiction needed to be treated first. They could have spent more time evaluating our son before taking our money, and now they are kicking him out.

Did they say to him, "We can't help you"? Now what? I'm furious. Breathe, Maria.

I call several dual treatment facilities, and every place sounds more depressing.

My son is not a criminal who needs to be locked up!

I leave five messages at treatment centers from Florida to Tennessee. My criteria for the right facility include a comfortable, home-like environment; guidance that will allow Josh to reach his highest level of independence; and psychotherapy to treat his depression with limited medication.

Finally, one night on my way home from work, I receive a callback from a very nice woman who's a director for a dual treatment place in Tennessee.

"Hello, this is Maria Martin," I say as I answer the phone.

"Hi, Ms. Martin, this is Beth Hall with the Smoky Mountain Lodge treatment center," she says with such kindness in her voice.

"Thank you for calling me back." I exhale.

"Of course. Please tell me about Josh," she asks me sincerely.

I start from the beginning and tell her everything.

"We can help Josh. Each resident has individual and group therapy. Everyone helps with everyday chores, such as serving meals and cleaning up. We have equine therapy and exercise programs. We will customize treatments to help Josh with his depression and addiction. I can call the North Carolina wilderness facility to coordinate meeting them halfway so we can bring Josh to Tennessee."

"How soon can your team meet the other director to bring Josh to your facility?" I ask.

"First thing on Monday—I can make that happen," she answers with confidence.

"OK," I hesitantly answer. "I agree to move Josh to your facility."

"Great, I will email the paperwork to you tomorrow."

I call Aaron to tell him about moving Josh.

"I honestly don't know how we are going to pay for this, Maria. My insurance doesn't cover all of it."

"We have to help our son," I respond, choking back my tears.

"I want to help him too," Aaron acquiesces. "I will call the wilderness facility tomorrow to discuss paying for the time Josh was there and getting a refund."

I am exhausted. *I feel sad for Josh. I just want real help for him. I pray this new place can make a difference for him.*

The following weekend, I will see Josh for the first time after seeing him at the hospital near Clemson. Aaron had more time off from work over the past month and was able to move Josh to North Carolina. Last week, the director of the new place met the director of the wilderness place and brought Josh to Tennessee. I know he's confused about moving from place to place. And he's probably still very angry at me.

God, please let this be the right place for Josh. I know he feels so alone.

It's a four-and-a-half-hour drive to Tennessee. I stop only once. I can't wait to see my son.

The facility is about fifteen minutes outside of Gatlinburg. The leaves are bright yellow, crimson red, and burnt orange—it's as if God painted the trees. Driving the winding road up the mountain, I can't help admiring the beauty of where Josh is staying. And at the same time, I realize he must feel like he's in yet another prison.

The building is made all of wood and looks like a resort. I park in the gravel driveway and walk up the steps onto the wraparound porch. Opening the door, I see patients reading and watching TV; one young man is even playing the piano. I'm greeted with a big smile from one of the nurses at the desk.

"Hi, I'm Maria Martin, Josh's mom," I announce to the director as she walks up to me.

"He's been looking forward to seeing you," she responds. "I will go get him."

Off she goes as I find a couch to sit on. Josh comes out, and I burst into tears. I stand up as he comes toward me. Josh gives me a big hug—he doesn't let go.

"Mom, I'm sorry I got upset with you. I'm so glad that you are here," he whispers through his tears.

"Me too, I love you." I hug my son tighter. "I forgive you."

"Would you like to have lunch with us?" Josh asks.

"I would love to." We walk into the dining room together.

It's family style, and all the patients are seated around the long, rectangular table. Handpicked sunflowers from their garden fill several blue pottery vases lined up along the center of the table. Lunch is baked chicken, green beans, mashed potatoes, fresh-baked rolls, and salad with carrots, celery, red onions, shredded cheddar cheese, and homemade croutons. The food is delicious and very healthy.

Thank you, God, for the good food and for such a nurturing place for Josh to heal.

Kevin, one of the other young men here, is very talkative. "So, you're from South Carolina? Is it nice there? Josh says it's near the beach. I've never been to the beach. Josh plays cards with me. He's very nice," Kevin says, all in one breath.

"Yes, we do live in Charleston, South Carolina, near the beach. I'm glad you and Josh are friends." Kevin smiles and returns to his food in front of him.

We all help by clearing our dishes. After lunch, Josh wants to show me around. There are trees and flowers surrounding the walkways and gardens with plenty of seating. My favorite tree is a gorgeous, bright red Japanese maple. We sit down on a bench near that beautiful tree, overlooking the mountains.

"Mom, you and Dad don't have to pay for such a fancy place for me," Josh tells me point-blank.

Thinking that he doesn't like it, I hesitate to respond. Then I realize that he feels unworthy.

"Josh, your father and I want you to be here. You deserve all of this, and you deserve to be happy and healthy." I look right at my wonderful son.

Josh looks back at me with tears in his eyes. I touch his hand, and we sit in silence.

Then he asks, "Mom, will I always feel depressed?"

I try to speak through the lump in my throat. "I promise to continue to help you to find the right care and medicine. I love you."

The time with him goes by too fast. I hate to leave him again. The center's policy is one afternoon visit per month. Luckily, I'm staying at a hotel overnight before I have to drive home.

"Josh, I love you so much."

"I love you, Mom."

I give him a big hug. *God, be with Josh. Please help him to heal.*

I get into my car and open my phone to check for any messages. I have one alert, a daily scripture. The scripture for the day, Psalm 121:8, says:

The Lord will keep
your going out and your coming in
from this time forth and forevermore.

I know the scripture is God's words for Josh.

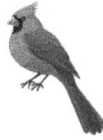

CHAPTER TWENTY

Temporary Calm

Josh

I realize when I wake up that it's Christmas Eve. One of the therapists knocks on my door to let me know that Dad is here. I want to go home, but I'm nervous too. I meet Dad in the lobby.

"Hey, Dad." I'm really happy to see him.

"Hi, Josh!" Dad looks just as happy to see me. He gives me a huge hug.

We have breakfast together; that includes eggs, grits, sausage links, homemade biscuits, and fresh-squeezed orange juice. I will miss the great food here. After breakfast, I head to my room to gather my stuff. I say goodbye to a few of the patients. Kevin hugs me hard—I will miss him the most. Dad's signing me out when I meet him back in the lobby. We head outside and put my backpack and suitcase in the car.

After two months, I have learned coping skills in therapy, and the medicine seems to be helping. My doctors agreed I could go home.

I look at my reflection in the side-view mirror. My eyes look tired and a little sad. I still have moments of sadness.

I want to tell Dad that as we head down the winding driveway.

I stay quiet because right now I'm happy to be going home.

"Josh, are you concerned about coming home?" Dad asks me. I really do think my parents can read my mind sometimes.

"Yes," I reply. "I'm also disappointed about not going back to college."

"Well, your mom and I will help you continue with the best treatment at home and also figure out when it's a good time for you to start college classes again."

"Thank you, Dad." I close my eyes. *Thank you, God, for my parents.*

When we get home, I take a long shower and put on clean clothes. We stopped for lunch on the way home, but it was a long ride, and I'm hungry again.

"Dad, what's good to eat?" I ask, walking into the kitchen.

"We can order a pizza. What kind would you like?" he asks.

"I would love a Hawaiian pizza," I request.

So, for Christmas Eve dinner, Dad and I have Hawaiian pizza. Dad keeps the conversation light, but he seems worried. We watch a little TV before I head to bed. Mom calls to say good night and that she can't wait to see me tomorrow.

Mom does love Christmas, and I know she has gifts for me too. That brings a smile to my face. Getting into bed, I quickly drift off to sleep.

I slept so well—it's Christmas morning. Dad made breakfast for us. Smelling the bacon and eggs, I realize how hungry I am again.

"Merry Christmas," Dad says as I walk out.

"Merry Christmas, Dad." I sit on a barstool at the kitchen counter.

Dad looks more relaxed. He smiles at me as he places my plate on the counter.

I'm happy to be back home, yet I feel anxious. Even around my family, I sometimes don't know what to say. I hope it will go away over time, but the anxiety is always there. And then the depression sneaks in.

My parents love me unconditionally. That should be enough, but I feel unworthy and then guilty for all they do. Sure, there are moments when I feel lighter, and sometimes even happy. Often, I get angry that nothing seems to help.

Mom and Dad are persistent, so I go along with it—going to the places they send me, seeing a psychiatrist, taking antidepressants.

I'm not trying to be deceptive. It's just easier to say I'm feeling better and agree that the medication and the therapists are helping me.

Ugh, why do I have to think like this on Christmas?

I clear my breakfast plate and head to the bathroom. I let the hot water wash away all the negative thoughts and feelings. After my shower, I find my green sweater, knowing that Mom will love my festive attire.

Oh, Carrie. I think of her just then. She finished fall semester at her college. I didn't get to visit her. I hope she forgives me. *I have been sick,* I want to tell her.

Is that true? No, not really. I will call and wish her a merry Christmas.

Dad hands me the keys to his car. "Here you go. See you later tonight."

"Thanks, Dad. I love you." I head to the garage and get in the car.

I hook my phone up to the Bluetooth in Dad's car. I dial Carrie's number.

"Hi, Carrie, I'm sorry I have not called you sooner. I just got home last night."

"Hi, Josh. Merry Christmas." Carrie is quiet. I'm sure she hates me. "Josh, I know you have been through a lot, but I just want you to be honest with me."

I'm quiet for a minute. *How can I be honest about how I feel?*

"OK, I'm afraid you won't like me anymore if I tell you that I'm severely depressed."

"Josh, thank you for sharing that with me. And of course I still like you. Can I see you when I get back home? I'm visiting family in Pennsylvania."

"Yes, I would like that very much," I say, really missing her now.

"See you when I get back. Enjoy your Christmas with your family."

"You too. Merry Christmas." I hang up the phone.

Happy New Year. I'm ready for a new and happy one.

"This year will be different," I say aloud as I get out of bed.

Last New Year's Day comes dreadfully to mind.

How could I have been so sad that I wanted to take my own life?

I'm happy to be home, but I still feel isolated from my friends. Dad and I talked the other night, and I'm going to enroll in the local community college. Going over to Mom's again today will be fun. Dad is still asleep, so I quietly close the front door and head out.

My younger brother and sister are up when I arrive.

"Hi, Audra. Hi, AJ," I announce with my arrival.

"Hi," they both reply as I'm greeted by Buddy. He's twelve and still acts like a puppy. He follows me as I go into the kitchen to see what Mom is doing.

"Hi, Josh." Mom smiles and hands me a biscuit.

"Hi, Mom. Thank you. This is really good," I say after taking a huge bite into the warm homemade biscuit.

Mom is cooking her traditional New Year's dinner of pork, sauerkraut, and (now that she considers herself a Southerner), Hoppin' John. I really have no idea how it got that name. It's made of flavorless beans and tastes worse than the sauerkraut. So, I will eat the pork, pass on both sides, and ask Mom for applesauce and more biscuits.

We all watch football while Mom is cooking, and I think about the silly tradition of New Year's resolutions. I've never had any New Year's resolutions.

What I desire seems bigger than that. *What do I do with my life now? I want to be here, but I want to feel better. I can't understand why I still feel this way.*

I talk to Dr. Allen about how I'm feeling, and sometimes I feel better after we talk. She's my therapist here in town. The medicine really doesn't help, and my sleep is always terrible. Sometimes I'm up all night, and then I sleep all day.

I don't know what to say to Carrie when we see each other. She will be home from Pennsylvania in a few days. I'll call her tomorrow.

"Dinner is ready," Mom shouts from the kitchen.

We gather around the dining room table. Mom says a quick prayer, and we eat.

"Josh, would you like applesauce with your pork?"

"Yes, thanks, Mom," I answer.

"AJ, do you want some Hoppin' John?"

"Yuck, Mom! Can I get more biscuits?" he says, making a face.

"Yes, of course." Mom chuckles, knowing her food traditions are strange. "Audra, how is your thesis coming along for school?"

"I just got the grant approved to work with the professor at the College of Charleston this summer," Audra shares with us.

"That's awesome, sweetheart," Mom responds.

"Mom, I have decided to take classes at the community college this spring," I chime in.

"Josh, that's really great to hear." I know Mom is proud of me too.

"I want to keep my education on track. And I want to start refereeing again. I know the exercise will be good for me, and the kids are the easiest to work with."

I remember being a kid and enjoying playing games, and just enjoying life. I know I still have a long way to go to feel like me again, but doing the things I love will help. I feel happier when I do the things I love and when I'm with my family.

"Mom, thanks for dinner and for today." I help Mom clear the table.

"You're welcome. I'm glad you enjoyed the day."

Mom invites me to watch a movie with her. Even though I've had a good day, I'm tired.

I decide to head to my room and get some sleep. But of course, I just lie there as sleep eludes me. Mom has kept everything the same in my childhood room. I sleep here when I visit her. Dad will be away for work, so I will be here for the next ten days. I will make the most of my time while I'm here with Mom.

Maybe Mom and I can visit the community college together.

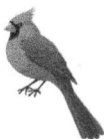

CHAPTER TWENTY-ONE

It's All Unraveling

Maria

During my lunch break at work, I look at pictures from Christmas. It was great having everyone home. I'm so thankful that Audra, Curt, and AJ always make Josh feel welcome, knowing how he's been feeling.

Just then the phone rings—it's Audra. She's out of breath.

"Mom, I think Josh took something!" she yells into the phone. "He's smashing things all over the house!"

"I'll be right home! Call your dad! He just got back from his work trip this morning. He's closer and can get there before me." I speak quickly, locking my computer and grabbing my purse.

No! Not again! I drive as fast as I can.

"911, what is your emergency?" the dispatcher asks me.

"My son has taken illegal drugs. He may be a danger to himself and his sister."

"What's your address, ma'am?"

I respond with our address, trying to speak through my sobs.

I hope Aaron will get to the house quickly.

And I pray that Josh and Audra will be OK.

When I arrive at the house, Aaron and the police are already there. Opening the front door, I see chairs knocked down, chips crushed into the carpet, and books thrown everywhere. Josh is in his room, yelling something I can't understand.

I head up the stairs, fearful of what I might find. Aaron is trying to calm Josh down.

I smell something metallic. I see blood on the bed and the carpet. Josh doesn't appear to be hurt, though. When I look into my bedroom, it's turned upside down. Sheets, bedspread, pillows, and the mattress thrown on the floor. All the picture frames and glass candlesticks on my dresser are smashed. Josh must have stepped on the broken glass covering the floor.

The police officer puts Josh in handcuffs. I hear them click into place. The officer sees the look of horror on my face. He explains to us that they're to prevent Josh from hurting himself further.

I hate seeing my son like this! Josh was doing so well. How can it spiral so quickly back to chaos? I shudder with the fear; Josh or Audra could have been seriously hurt.

An ambulance arrives, and the paramedics meet the police officer. I start to cry again as they escort Josh to the ambulance. Once the paramedics leave to take him to the hospital, the officer asks to talk to us.

"We have to search the house since there were illegal drugs here, and Josh took them on the premises," the officer explains as kindly as he can. "Mrs. Martin, you can leave since you arrived after me." He detains Audra and Aaron and searches the house.

I head to the hospital and wait to see Josh. The doctor comes out to talk to me. He agrees to let me see my son. They have him restrained in the bed. Tears well up in my eyes as I walk toward the bed he is lying on. Josh looks at me but doesn't recognize me as his mom.

I put my hand on top of his. "I love you, Josh." *I hope he knows how much I love him.*

Josh gets very agitated, and the doctor tells me it's probably best to let him rest. He needs to safely detox again. I leave him in the doctor's care.

Once again, I'm in my car, crying and yelling. "God, please show me how to help my son. I hate seeing him in so much pain. Heal him of this horrible disease. Depression is a monster that is slowly killing my son!" I scream and slam my fists onto the steering wheel. I cry all the way home.

We all clean up the house in silence. When Aaron leaves, I go to Audra's room first.

"You OK?" I ask my very brave daughter.

"Yes, Mom," she whispers.

"I'm proud of you for being courageous," I say with so much love. "You saved Josh's life."

"Mom, he was just messed up with drugs," Audra shares.

"I know, but he could have hurt himself. You protected him by talking to him and calling us for help. I will do everything I can to keep you from having to experience that again," I tell her. But I really have no control of my adult son.

I go to check on AJ, even though he was at track tryouts with his friend earlier.

"Mom, will Josh get better?" he asks.

"I hope so," I respond, being as upbeat as I can. I hug him and say, "Good night. Sleep well."

Once again, I'm lying on my bed and staring up at the ceiling.

How can we as a family be fine when Josh is in so much pain? Will he get better? Will he continue to bring harm to himself? This time he could have hurt his sister too. How can I really keep him from harm? Do I find another facility so he can receive around-the-clock help?

The officer found a postage stamp–size square pouch containing the LSD powder that Josh took.

God, please show me how to help my son.

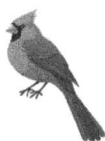

CHAPTER TWENTY-TWO

White Walls and Restraints

I'm so tired of being here ...

And if you have to leave

I wish that you would just leave

'Cause your presence still lingers here ...

These wounds won't seem to heal, this pain is just too real

—"My Immortal," Evanescence

Josh

I wake up. I'm strapped to the bed. I try to move. Ow, the straps are really tight. I look around. I see a guard sitting by the door.

What the hell happened?

Oh. Yeah. I took LSD and went crazy.

Oh, no! I trashed Mom's house. It must look pretty bad.

Ugh, I feel terrible. I feel sweat dripping down my back. I start shaking violently again.

A nurse comes in to put something in my IV. It relaxes me, and I drift off.

When I wake up, it's dark outside again.

How long have I been here? Why didn't I remember how awful it feels to detox?

Somebody, help me.

My feelings start to come back. *Why am I crying? I'm really sad now.*

Can someone help me with my depression? I don't want to take drugs. They make me feel better. And help me to forget everything.

I am freezing.

The nurse comes in again, and she brings me another blanket and a fresh pillow. The pillow she removes from under my head is soaking wet. She knew I needed another blanket too.

It's light outside again. I slept through the night. A new nurse comes in.

"Are you hungry?" she asks me.

"No," I respond, "I'm really thirsty." I drink three Gatorades, and I'm still thirsty.

Was Mom here? Yes, she was here when the first nurse was here. Now, two nurses later, my family has still not come back. Right when I have that negative thought, Mom walks through the door.

"Hi, Josh," she greets me.

"Hi, Mom." I look away.

"How are you?" she asks me.

"I've been better," I grunt.

Mom pauses, gathering her courage to talk to me. "I'm going to have a quick word with the doctor."

As she turns to open the door, the doctor walks in. He looks distracted, and Mom doesn't ask him any questions.

"Be sure to get lots of fluids and rest," the doctor finally says to me.

What? I don't have a cold. I took LSD!

The doctor leaves the room, and Mom turns to look at me. "Well, that doctor is not helpful at all. Let's go home."

"OK, Mom." I want to tell her I'm sorry. But I really don't want to talk about it.

It's weeks later; I can't sleep at all now. Before, I could sleep during the day; now I only sleep for a few hours at night and not at all during the day. Daisy, Dad's cat, sits with me and sleeps with me too. I talk to her throughout the day. She follows me everywhere. Dad says she is my cat now.

I do like her company. Snoops, his other cat, ignores me completely.

I had agreed to take classes at the local technical college, but now I don't want to go.

Classes start in two weeks. We just bought my books. I'm only taking two classes this semester. Dad's leaving tomorrow morning, and he will be back from his work trip by then. His place is closer to the campus than Mom's.

"Dinner is ready!" Dad yells from the kitchen.

"Be right there." I get up off my bed and walk to the kitchen.

Dad made steak and potatoes. I'm starving and dive right into my steak.

"What time are you leaving tomorrow, Dad?"

"My flight is at noon." Dad looks up.

"I will head over to Mom's around eleven o'clock tomorrow morning."

"Don't forget to come to feed the cats three times a week."

"I will, Dad," I answer between bites.

The worst part about going to Mom's will be driving back and forth. They're trusting me with the car but not with my medication or to stay by myself. Mom picked up my prescriptions yesterday to have at her place. I really want to still be at college and on my own. I wish that I had not taken so many drugs that night. Then I would not be where I am now. I had taken Xanax a few times in high school, but that was the first time I took LSD.

Taking drugs is one thing I can control. I feel out of control with my feelings and everything else. Depression just follows me everywhere. It's an evil demon that invades my mind all day and all night. It invades my body, preventing sleep and making me tired all the time. It invades my heart; I feel sadness in every part of my body. I just want to hide sometimes. Other times I want to feel better with drugs or pot. And then, sometimes, I want it all to just end.

I share my thoughts with Dr. Allen, and she reassures me that I can always reach out for help.

Help with what? I'm so stuck in my mind and body that I want to escape.

I never feel better. I have felt this way since my concussion when I was twelve.

Some of my friends have stopped calling and texting me. I don't blame them. I sound depressing. Alec texts me sometimes.

Carrie still calls and texts me, but I still have not gone to see her or asked her to come see me. When she got back from Pennsylvania, I was in the hospital again. I wouldn't blame her if she moved on.

I do still love her. I have always loved her. Deep down, I know that she loves me too.

So here comes the courage again. I will ask Carrie to visit when I'm at Mom's house. It's closer to her. She and my mom get along well. Mom can fill in the silence when I don't have anything to say.

I will ask Mom if Carrie can visit next week. I know she will agree and be excited that I'm reaching out again.

But even when I want to see Carrie one moment, I don't the next. *What would our relationship be like if I were normal?*

Carrie says she loves me just as I am. My thoughts go back to that perfect beach day.

I felt normal. I was me that day.

I pick up my cell phone to text her. *Hi.*

Hi, Carrie texts back immediately.

I will be at Mom's house next week. Would you like to come for dinner?

I would love to.

OK, let me confirm with Mom, even though we both know she will say yes. I send a smiley emoji.

Just let me know which day is best.

I will. I miss you, I text her.

I miss you too, she texts right back.

Good night. Sleep well.

Good night, Josh. You too.

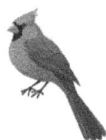

CHAPTER TWENTY-THREE

New Courage

Maria

I wake up feeling exhausted. But I'm so excited. Grant and I are going to a Prince tribute concert tonight. I walk into my closet and try on a few outfits. I choose black jeans, a shimmery silver blouse, and black wedges. After my yoga video, I spend an hour and a half in the bathroom. It's wonderful taking a luxurious bubble bath. I give myself a pedicure, painting my toenails my favorite shade of red.

AJ is with his dad and is spending time with Josh too. And Audra is working on a school project and spending the night with her best friend, Sarah. I finally venture downstairs to have coffee. My back porch is my favorite place. I enjoy the rest of my morning reading.

My mind wanders to Grant; I'm looking forward to our conversations and kisses tonight.

Grant calls just then. "Morning, beautiful. Can't wait to see you tonight. Can I pick you up at six o'clock?"

"Hi, morning. I'm very excited to see you too. Yes, six o'clock is perfect. See you then." After hanging up the phone, I can't stop smiling.

I have several hours before Grant comes to pick me up. I pick up the phone to call Josh and see how he's doing.

"Hi, how are you?" I ask him when he answers the phone.

"A little better. Mom, I'm so sorry. I broke your picture frames and candlesticks and made an awful mess."

"I forgive you. What happened?" I ask him.

"On New Year's Day, all of the memories from the previous year came back. And each day, I would get more and more agitated and upset. I ordered the LSD using Bitcoin and had it sent to the house."

"Josh, your dad is going on another trip. Do you think you can avoid doing drugs?"

"I promise I will not buy any more drugs. And I'll go to see my therapist next week," Josh says in response to my question.

"Josh, please keep your promise." I'm really nervous about having him home again but keep that to myself. "Enjoy your day. I love you."

I go inside to put my coffee cup away. I put on jeans and a sweater and head out to the grocery store. AJ, Audra, and Josh will be here tomorrow. I need to restock the refrigerator and pantry before they come home.

Once I've unloaded the groceries, I finish folding the clothes in the dryer. I always gravitate to chores when I'm nervous—I'm still thinking about Josh.

I will tell Grant what happened with Josh another day; tonight is just for us.

"Enough," I say out loud. Pouring myself a glass of rosé, I put on Led Zeppelin. I head back upstairs to spend more time pampering myself. I pull out my hot rollers and plug them in.

Dancing around my bathroom with rollers in my hair makes me laugh. I finish putting on my makeup and get dressed in the outfit

I chose this morning. Adding earrings, my rings, and my favorite perfume, I'm finally ready.

The doorbell rings. *He's here.* I feel like a teenager running down the stairs.

Opening the door with a huge smile, I simply say, "Hello."

"You look wonderful." Grant smiles at me.

"Thank you. You look pretty good too." Grant looks so handsome in jeans and a navy button-down shirt. "Give me a second to grab my purse."

As I turn to head back inside, Grant grabs my hand and spins me around. He kisses me so passionately, time simply stops. I blush, and he smiles again.

"You ready to go?" he asks playfully.

"I am," I respond with a laugh.

We decide to eat again at our favorite restaurant, Halls.

"Thank you for the concert tickets," Grant adds to the conversation.

"You're welcome—it should be a fun concert."

We walk from the restaurant to the Charleston Music Hall. The ushers scan our tickets, and we go to find our seats.

"Would you like a glass of wine?" Grant turns to me.

"Yes—red, please," I respond with a wink.

"Be right back." Grant leans in to kiss me before he leaves.

While Grant is gone, fear creeps in. *Josh is fine. Breathe, Maria.* I breathe in and out slowly. *Josh will be fine tonight. I can enjoy the concert.*

The concert is so much fun. Our seats are at the end of the row, and we dance in the aisle all throughout the concert. Grant knows every song and sings out loud. I laugh and sing along with him. I love seeing him be himself around me.

Hand in hand, we leave the music hall. We search for a cool bar to have a nightcap in. The bar we find close by is called Prohibition.

I love the names of their various drinks. I decide to have a simple old-fashioned, after changing my mind several times. Grant has his favorite drink: tequila on the rocks.

After our drinks, we walk around downtown Charleston for a while, simply enjoying each other's company before heading home.

"Would you like to come in?" I boldly ask Grant at my front door. I want him to come in, even though I know it may be too soon.

"I would love to, but I may not want to leave."

I smile and nod. He kisses me again, more passionately than before.

"Thank you for a wonderful evening, Maria." Grant looks right into my eyes.

"Thank you. Good night," I say, blushing.

"Good night, beautiful."

I wake up this morning with a sinking feeling, and all the worry has returned. Josh has been staying with his dad. We're both concerned about him. We don't want him taking drugs, and yet he is on three different drugs to help him with his depression and sleep. Aaron is going away for work for a week, and Josh will be staying with me again.

Why does something always happen when he stays with me?

I work in private wealth, supporting a financial advisor and his clients. I've made arrangements and have been granted time off so that I can work part-time when Josh is with me and be off a few days too. That way I can be around to keep an eye on him. I hate that I have to babysit my nineteen-year-old son, but I really don't know what else to do. He will be coming over later this morning when his dad leaves for the airport. I'm anxious and cleaning his room for the third time.

I head downstairs to start my coffee. Just as I turn off the coffeepot, Josh comes in the front door. He seems nervous to be home too.

"Hi, Josh, I'm glad you're here." *I will be brave; I do want my son here.*

"Me too, Mom." Josh looks defeated.

"Would you like scrambled eggs for breakfast?" I ask.

"Yeah, sounds good." Josh regains some courage.

"So, you start class in a few weeks?" I ask as I beat the eggs with a whisk.

"Yeah, Dad got my books this week."

"You excited or concerned about going back?" I question.

"A little of both." Josh looks apprehensive.

We eat breakfast mostly in silence. I clear our breakfast plates. "You can go upstairs and get settled in your room."

"OK, I will." Josh heads upstairs.

I decide to wait until later, during dinner, to ask him the tougher questions. *Is he still feeling depressed? Has he been having suicidal thoughts? How's it going with him and his dad?* I feel sad just thinking about Josh still being depressed.

I distract myself by heading into the garage in search of gardening tools. Being in the South, it can be really warm in early February. Today, it's seventy degrees. I find my shovel and spade and gloves. I start working on the back flower beds, clearing out dead leaves and weeds.

Working with my hands in the dirt really helps to calm me. I feel such peace and a connection with nature.

Just as I finish clearing the first flower bed, Josh comes outside.

"Hi, Mom. Need any help?" he asks me.

"Sure, I would love some help." I tell him where to find more gloves and the rake, and we both start pulling weeds from the second flower bed—the vegetable garden that's been abandoned for years.

Working in silence next to my son, clearing years of neglect, is very cathartic.

"Josh, thank you for doing this with me." I look up and wipe my brow.

"I actually like working outside like this." Josh is smiling.

I smile to myself. "Me too, Josh."

Two hours later, we both stand up simultaneously.

"I'm going to go take a shower and then start dinner," I tell him.

"I will put the spade, gloves, and shovel away," Josh offers.

"We are having burgers for dinner." I hand him my gloves.

"Sounds great, Mom."

I go upstairs to take a super hot shower. The temperature dropped while we were outside. I put on my favorite yoga pants and a cashmere sweater.

"I'm done in the shower," I tell Josh, and then I head downstairs.

I busy myself in the kitchen to distract me from my thoughts.

How did I go from feeling so connected to my son to my mind spinning again?

I definitely want to ask Josh how he's feeling. *God, please give me the courage and the words to ask Josh how he's feeling.*

As I set the table, I hear Josh get into the shower. I put on some music—Frank Sinatra is the best music to relax me.

AJ will be home from a track meet later tonight, so Josh and I will have time to talk during dinner.

"Josh, dinner's ready," I announce twenty minutes later.

"Be right down."

Josh looks more relaxed. We enjoy a simple meal of hamburgers, fries, and a salad.

"Can I get you more to drink?" I motion to the pitcher of iced tea.

"No, Mom, although I do love your iced tea." He pauses. "Mom, I want to thank you."

"What for, Josh?"

I see tears fill his eyes. "Everything." He pauses. "You and Dad have done so much for me."

"You're so welcome. I want you to know that we will always be here for you."

"I know," he whispers.

"Josh, how have you been feeling?" I finally ask him.

"I feel sad and alone a lot," he shares with me.

"I'm sorry." I choke back my tears.

Then I just cry, realizing that the best thing to do is feel and show Josh he can feel sad too. A single tear falls down my son's cheek. And then another. He doesn't brush them away. I reach out to hold his hand, and we sit in the silence with our feelings. Several minutes pass, and I realize that words are not necessary now. Josh gets up and starts clearing the table. He's like me in that—sometimes it's comforting to be busy rather than being with your feelings. We clean up in silence; however, we are together.

I want to tell him that everything is going to be OK and that he will feel better soon. To be honest, I know that I'm not able to give him that reassurance. But I still want to give him hope.

"Josh, I know that I cannot fix everything for you. But I will continue to help."

"I know, Mom, and that means a lot." He looks away.

"I know that this house holds a lot of memories for you," I continue.

"Yeah, but I also know things are different now." My wise son really does know.

"Are you having any thoughts?" I question him.

"I have not been having any suicidal thoughts," he quickly answers.

"How have you been sleeping?" I ask him.

"Not great. I think I may head up to bed now."

"I love you." I hope he truly knows how much I love him.

"I love you too, Mom."

As I put the final dishes in the dishwasher, Audra and AJ come home at the same time.

"You both hungry?" I ask them.

"Yeah, Mom," Audra says.

I pull out the food I had just put away. After warming it up, I invite them both to eat.

"How was your day?" I ask, curious about both of them.

"It was good. I placed second in the 800, and we won the relay," AJ responds.

"Sorry I missed your meet. I am planning to go to the one next weekend," I tell him.

"It's all right. The meet was two hours away, and I always have to ride with the team on the bus. The next meet is at our high school."

"Great, I can definitely make that," I tell him.

"Thanks for the burger, Mom. I'm going to take a shower and then chill in my room." AJ puts his dish in the dishwasher and heads upstairs.

"You're welcome, AJ." Turning to my daughter, I ask her, "Audra, how did your studying go?"

"It went well—we're working on our senior project together," she responds.

"Are you getting excited about graduation?" I continue asking her about school.

"Yeah, I am. I'm ready to graduate."

"We can go dress shopping next weekend for both your prom and graduation dresses."

CHAPTER TWENTY-THREE

"That would be great, Mom. I want a short black dress for graduation," Audra adds.

"Any idea on what color you want for your prom dress? I think you would look beautiful in a navy dress." I'm excited for both her prom and graduation.

"That might work. Is Josh here?" Audra asks with concern.

"Yes, he helped me clean up the backyard for two hours this afternoon. He went to bed right before you both got home."

"How is he, Mom?" Audra looks at me questioningly.

"I think he is doing better, but he's still sad," I share.

"I'm worried about him. What if something happens again?" Audra tears up.

"I am too. But the medicine is helping him more this time."

Audra doesn't look convinced.

"And I'm working from home for the next two weeks. So, I will be here," I continue.

"OK. I'm still scared he may take drugs again." Audra gets up from the table.

I don't know what else to say to my daughter to reassure her.

"Would you like to watch a movie with me tonight?" I ask.

"I'm pretty tired, Mom. I think I'm just going to head to bed."

"OK, sleep well." Audra heads upstairs, and I clean up the kitchen again. I decide not to watch a movie; instead, I head upstairs.

"Good night, AJ. I'm heading to bed," I say to him while standing at his bedroom door.

"Good night, Mom."

I peek into Josh's room. He looks so peaceful sleeping. I close his door quietly and head to my room. Feeling restless, I decide to take a hot bubble bath to relax me. I turn on the faucet and fill the tub with hot water and my favorite lavender bubble bath. I pull up my

129

hair in a twist. After washing my face, I put on a clay mask. I grab a fluffy towel and slip into the bubbly water. I brought up the rest of my red wine from dinner. It's the perfect combination of relaxation for me. The day was long and challenging in many ways. However, Josh and I did have good conversations, and I enjoyed his company and his help with the backyard.

God, please be with all of us this week, I pray as I get out of the tub and dry off.

I open my bedside table to pull out my silk eye mask, and a card my mom sent me catches my eye. The words on the front of the card, from Psalm 31:24, are just what I needed to see.

"Be strong and take heart, all you who hope in the Lord."

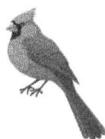

CHAPTER TWENTY-FOUR

Running Away

Josh

I've been with Mom almost a week. To be honest, it's not too bad this time. And I have finally been sleeping.

"Josh, you want breakfast?" Mom yells from the bottom of the stairs.

"Yes, be down after I take a shower." Heading to the bathroom, I take a quick shower.

I can't remember the last time I took one. Oh right, the day I got here. It's been four days. Guess I'm still feeling depressed.

The other reason why I want to take a shower is that Carrie is coming to dinner. I invited her earlier in the week, when I was feeling courageous.

I'm not feeling that way now.

Mom's making lasagna for dinner. She knows I love it. I'm sure Carrie will too.

After drying off, I wrap the towel around my waist and look in the mirror. I still look like I did in high school.

I just feel incredibly different now.

It's hard to find a clean shirt and shorts in my bag. I'll have to do some laundry after breakfast. Mom made chocolate chip pancakes. She's going all out today.

"Mom, the pancakes are delicious," I tell her after the first bite.

"Glad you like them." Mom smiles.

"And thank you for making lasagna for dinner tonight."

"You're very welcome," she replies with a wink.

After breakfast, I head back upstairs to do laundry. While I'm waiting for my dark clothes to finish washing, I open up my closet. This room was my room from elementary school through high school. The closet holds so many of my memories.

All of my soccer trophies are perched on the top shelf. They are next to all the sweaters that Dad gave me. He wore them when he was in high school up North. Although we live in the South, I wear them sometimes through the fall and winter. In a white plastic bag is my graduation cap and gown. I also have many Hawaiian shirts that I have acquired over the years. Some were given to me, but most of them I bought at Goodwill. I pull out several that I like and will still wear. Next to the Hawaiian shirts are long-sleeved button-down shirts in various colors. Mom bought the entire rainbow.

I pull out the pink one, my favorite. And there are my khaki pants, in various sizes as I grew over the years. After trying several on, I find two pairs that still fit me. I will wash the pink shirt, the khaki pants, and several Hawaiian shirts.

I transfer my dark clothes to the dryer and start the new load. I lie down in bed, waiting for my laundry.

When I wake up, the clock says it's four o'clock in the afternoon. I jump up and pull my dark clothes out of the dryer. I put the load from the washer into the dryer. While waiting for those clothes to dry, I take another shower.

Carrie will be here at six o'clock this evening. I want to look good.

I shave after my shower and use the cologne I find in my dresser. Pulling the clothes out of the dryer, I put on the pink shirt and a pair of the khakis. I have not dressed up in quite a while.

I'm very excited to see Carrie.

I find Mom in the kitchen, taking the lasagna out of the oven.

"Can I help?" I ask her.

"Sure, can you set the table? The napkins, silverware, and plates are on the dining room table." Mom turns around as she answers me. "Oh, you look very nice."

"Thanks." I walk into the dining room.

Mom has made garlic bread and salad to go with the lasagna.

"Carrie should be here any minute," I announce.

Just then, the doorbell rings. Now I'm really nervous. I head toward the front door.

"Hi," Carrie greets me immediately. She looks amazing in a pretty blue dress.

"You look great," I say. "Come in."

She enters the foyer, and I follow behind her to the kitchen.

"Hi, Mrs. Martin. How are you?" Carrie asks Mom.

"I'm good. How are you, Carrie?" Mom asks.

"I'm doing well. Thanks for having me to dinner."

"You're so welcome. It's great to see you."

We all sit down around the table. Mom serves the lasagna and says the blessing. The food's delicious, and I have seconds. So does Carrie. We talk and laugh. Mom asks Carrie a thousand questions about school. I have questions for her, but I want to wait until we are alone.

After we help Mom clean up, Carrie and I go out on the back porch together.

"Your mom was very inquisitive tonight," Carrie says right away.

"Yes, sorry about that," I reply sheepishly.

"I understand. She's always very talkative."

"Yes, she is." I laugh.

We sit in silence for a while. Carrie reaches over to hold my hand.

"Carrie, I realize you have a whole new life at school. And you may be seeing other people too. I may not like it, but I understand," I blurt out.

Carrie continues to hold my hand. "Josh, I will always love you. And I will always be here for you."

More silence.

I decide to make it easier for both of us. Because I realize she's better off finding someone who is happy.

"We can just be friends," I say, and I feel my heart drop to the floor.

Carrie starts to cry. I'm not sure if she is crying because she is sad or relieved.

"Josh, it's only been you in my life. Yes, I've made friends, but I'm not dating anyone."

I let the air out that I have been holding in. "I appreciate that, but I know that I'm different from when we first met."

"Yes," she sighs.

"And this is the hardest thing I've ever had to do. I have a lot of healing to do, and I can't expect you to wait for me to feel better."

Carrie continues to cry and hold my hand. "Are you sure?"

"Yes." But I'm not sure. I feel such a pain in my heart, I cannot breathe.

CHAPTER TWENTY-FOUR

That's when I know that I will always love her.

Carrie and I sit in silence for a while, just holding hands. We both don't want this moment to end. After what seems like an hour, we both stand up at the same time. We hug, and I cry this time. I walk her to the front door.

"Josh," Carrie whispers.

"Yes," I answer, not wanting to hear what she's going to say.

"I will miss you."

"I will miss you too."

Carrie pauses, and then she continues. "And I will always love you."

"I will always love you too." I know that's the only true thing I've said all night.

Carrie walks to her car, and I watch her drive away. It takes me several minutes before I can walk back inside.

That was one of the hardest things that I ever had to do, but I know it was the right decision.

For her.

For us.

But was it the best decision for me?

I go straight to my room and plop down onto my bed. I stare at the ceiling for the longest time. There are no feelings left in me. Then I start to sob: big, chest-heaving sobs. I cry myself to sleep.

I wake up at three in the morning, and I stare at the ceiling once again.

The pain in my heart is still there. I want to call Carrie and say I made a mistake.

But what I want more is to be the me I was when we were first together. *I don't know that me anymore.*

I start crying again. Mom always says that tears can heal. She can say some silly things. I don't feel that my tears are healing. If anything, I just feel more pain.

At least I am feeling something.

When I wake up again, it's seven in the morning. Getting out of bed, I put on my running shorts and my favorite Duke T-shirt. I carry my running shoes downstairs. After putting on my shoes, I head out the front door to run and clear my head. I easily remember the running paths and trails in my old neighborhood.

It's awesome to run when very few people are even awake yet. I see several deer, egrets, and even a great blue heron.

I feel close to nature and to God. It feels great to just run.

I want all the pain, anger, sadness, fear, and depression to disappear, and during my run, it seems to vanish.

I forget about the day-to-day struggle. *I feel free. I feel like the old me. I am happy.*

When I circle back and run back toward my street, it all returns. Back at the house, I climb the stairs, and I take a long, hot shower.

After I dry off, I put on a clean shirt and shorts. I crawl into bed and go back to sleep.

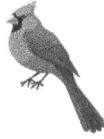

CHAPTER TWENTY-FIVE

Beautiful Storm

Maria

It's a beautiful spring day, and the water is crystal clear. My Mother's Day gift is kayaking with my kids. It took a little persuading to get everyone to go. However, once we walk down to the dock, Audra, AJ, and Josh all seem excited. Audra gets in a kayak with me. AJ and Josh go together.

Dolphins swim all around us. Herons and seagulls and egrets grace the water and the marshes. The water is so calm. It's a perfect day to be on the water.

We paddle out toward the Charleston Harbor. The waterway gets busier with paddleboarders, boaters, and fellow kayakers. Audra and I decide to follow the boys and get out to explore the marshes. Getting back in the kayak, we take on a good bit of water. I use my water bottle to empty some of it from the kayak. Heading toward Crab Bank island, I know we can't get out and walk because it's bird mating season, and stopping to explore the island would result in a fine. So, we start kayaking around it and then head back toward Shem Creek.

I notice the sky is getting darker. It starts to drizzle, and the wind picks up a little. We have a long way to go to get back to the dock.

As we come around the other side of the island, the sky falls out.

We're paddling so hard, but it seems like Audra and I are not moving forward. The tide is taking us out into the Charleston Harbor.

"Mom, what do we do?" Audra yells.

"We all need to go back toward the inlet," I shout so the boys can hear me too.

Audra and I paddle toward the inlet. The boys turn around to head our way, but they seem to be struggling too.

"AJ, everything OK?" I ask my youngest son.

"We're coming, Mom." I look back and see AJ paddling hard.

Josh seems to be very flustered.

"Audra, we have to turn around."

"Why, Mom? What's wrong with Josh?"

"Josh looks panicked, and he's having a hard time."

Audra and I turn the kayak around and head toward the boys. The rain is coming down harder, and visibility is terrible. I'm wiping water from my eyes with my drenched shirtsleeve. We're both getting tired, but I'm determined to get back to my boys.

"How are you doing?" I yell out to Josh and AJ.

They don't answer at first. When we finally reach them, Josh looks up at me.

"Just had a flashback and froze," he shares as he shudders.

"We're here to help." Our kayaks are now side by side. I try to remain calm so my kids do too. *Breathe, Maria.*

"Mom, just you coming back means a lot." Josh grips his paddle.

The boys start paddling together. My arms are burning now with the strain of paddling in the tumultuous water.

After what seems to be forever, we make it back into the mouth of the creek. We're not there yet, but we are closer. After ten more minutes of paddling, we finally reach the dock and climb out of our kayaks, soaked through. We all teeter on the dock.

I hug Audra and then AJ. Walking over to Josh, I give him a big hug too.

"What happened?" I ask him.

"I had a flashback about when I was a kid and Grandpa took me kayaking. The kayak tipped over, and Grandpa was there to rescue me. I didn't know if I would be strong enough to save AJ."

"I know you would have helped AJ. That's why it's important to go together."

"Love you, Josh," AJ says as he walks over and hugs his brother.

"Let's go dry off and get some hot chocolate," I offer to my children.

"Yes," all three of them say in unison.

What an incredible experience, though. From perfect beauty to black skies, with grit and love throughout. I will always remember this day.

I pray that my kids will remember this day too.

Especially Josh. I hope he knows that his family will be with him as he battles his depression.

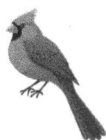

CHAPTER TWENTY-SIX

Terrible Thoughts

I'm going under ...
I got so used to the way you pulled me down ...
Still holding on to something lost ...
It breaks my heart but I can't stop
Holding on
—"Still Holding On," Jonathan Roy

Josh

I miss my friends and the fun. School was easy. The depression just got in the way. Being home for months, I feel more depressed than ever.

I aced both classes that I took during the second term of the spring semester. Living with Dad has been OK. We talk some, but recently I feel like we are roommates and not really father and son. Dad asks me all the time to go do things with him. I always say no. I really don't like socializing with other people, especially adults.

The only other person I talk to besides my family is my psychiatrist. I tell her a lot, but I haven't told her that the suicidal thoughts are back. I hate talking about having terrible thoughts of ending my life.

I'm sleeping all the time again. It's awful living this way. My parents are supportive, but they really don't understand. They want me to get better and be happy and healthy, but I feel worse every day.

What would be the easiest way to go? I hate having these thoughts, but I can't stop them.

Dad is around a lot; however, he does go out with his friends sometimes at night.

So, I begin to think about how ... and when ... and where to end it all.

Today is the longest day of my life. I spend most of it in bed.
Thinking.
Waiting.
Listening to music.
I fall asleep. I wake up. I realize it is dark out. I turn on the lamp.
Dad knocks on my door. "Josh, I'm heading to the concert now. Sure you don't want to come with me?"

"I'm good. Bye, Dad."

"Bye, Josh."

Dad leaves the house. That may be the last time I hear those words from him.

I take out my pot and smoke off and on for half an hour. I want to feel numb, but not too numb. Actually, I smoke for an hour. I look around the room one more time.

I see the picture of the bridge I took to college. I remember how fun it was at college.

I go to my closet to get my shoes. I grab the car keys.

I don't even say goodbye to the cats.

I go out the front door and down the back stairway. I unlock the car door and get in and sit for a while.

Then I start driving toward Charleston. I turn the radio on and then turn it off.

I don't remember the drive at all—just that there were very few cars on the road.

I park the car on the side of the road. I just leave the keys.

Then I walk slowly up the path toward the bridge. I look to see who's around.

No one is on the bridge.

It's about eleven o'clock at night. I can hear fireworks in the distance, even though it's only July 2.

I continue walking to the top of the bridge.

Once at the top, I stop. I cannot see beyond the side of the bridge.

I climb over the railing. I turn around. I pause, still holding on.

I feel fear.

Then I don't feel anything.

I close my eyes.

And I let go.

I had a dream—or was it a dream? In my dream, I sit in the car for a while.

Then I drive to the park near the bridge.

I get out of the car and walk up the pedestrian path on one side of the bridge. Once I get to the top, I stop. I look out over the edge. I remember hearing fireworks.

I am standing on the side of the bridge, holding on.

I feel fear.

I let go.

My mind goes blank.

I feel free.

Then I hit the water.

Ow, that really hurts! Did I break my bones? It feels like a thousand knives stabbing my chest and my lungs. *It feels so awful.* I start moving my arms. Then kick my legs to get above the water.

Everything hurts now. My eyes start to swell up, and it gets harder to see.

I start swimming, but my arms hurt so badly.

I stop swimming. *Oh, I can float.*

Then I swim again until it hurts.

Will I make it to the shore? Will I drown anyway?

I want to live. God, please help me.

Every movement hurts, but I don't stop swimming. I see something up ahead. Or is it my mind playing tricks on me?

It's a dock. I'm sure of it. I swim a little faster.

I finally reach the dock. I hold on with both arms over the edge, but I'm too weak to pull myself up.

I cry out for help. But there is no one around. Between my cries for help, I drift off.

I wake up because of the intense pain. I cry out one more time.

I hear a guy's voice. "Look, there's a young man hanging on the dock over there."

"Is he hurt?" a female voice responds.

CHAPTER TWENTY-SIX

The voices get closer. Am I dreaming that the two people can hear and see me?

"My name is Josh. I'm going to pull you up slowly," the male voice says. We have the same first name.

I don't remember if I said anything. I only remember being lifted up by these people.

I hear a siren.

Then everything goes dark.

It wasn't a dream.

I'm in another hospital bed. This time the physical pain is worse than the emotional pain. Every part of my body hurts. And I'm still not able to see.

When I hit the water, the pain was excruciating. I remember gasping for air as the water poured into my lungs. I struggled to breathe and to stay above water.

I was alive though. And I recall that a peace washed over me.

It was then that I chose to swim.

I chose to live.

I still feel numb, but I want to be happy again.

My dream was real.

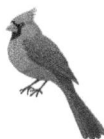

CHAPTER TWENTY-SEVEN

The Bridge

Maria

I wake up very disoriented, squinting at my phone. I see it's 1:03 a.m., and I have several missed calls from Aaron.

Audra is in my bedroom, waking me up. "It's Dad. On the phone," she says, handing me her phone. "Mom, wake up!"

Aaron is very upset. "Josh is gone. I went to a concert." He catches his breath. "When I got back, he wasn't here. He took the car!"

My mind tries to make sense of what Aaron is saying and wake up. "I'm going to call the detective." This was the same detective who helped us when Josh was in middle school. "I'll call you back." The detective doesn't answer, so I call Aaron back.

He is crying. "Josh is in the ER. Maria, Josh jumped! From the Charleston Bridge!"

Somehow, I calmly say, "I will be right there to pick you up."

Inside, I'm screaming, *NO! NOT AGAIN! OH NO! OH NO! OH NO!*

How did he survive? How is he alive after that jump?

I am sobbing as I drive to pick up Aaron, who had too much to drink at the concert to be able to drive himself.

Why, Josh? Why? I scream.

When I pick Aaron up, he's still crying. And I am in shock. We are both quiet during the drive. By the grace of God, I drive us safely to the hospital.

We walk into the hospital. I don't remember checking in at the front desk. I only remember Aaron's hand shaking as he pushes open the large metal door to the ER.

Nothing could have prepared me to see my son lying in the ER bed. He looks like a truck hit him. Both his eyes are swollen shut. He has bruises and cuts all over his body. My tears start flowing.

I turn to grab hold of the shelves behind me so I won't fall. I feel so sick to my stomach. I'm sure I am going to pass out. I start hyperventilating. *Breathe, Maria. Breathe.*

God, please give me courage. God, please help me. God, please help my son.

I walk over to the bed Josh is lying on. I lean over to kiss his forehead.

"Josh, I love you so much," I tell him, over and over and over again, while I hold his hand.

My son jumped the equivalent of eighteen stories and landed on his face and stomach. He fractured his cheekbones and eye sockets and his right clavicle. He has bruises and contusions all over his body. He has no internal bleeding or paralysis. The doctors go on to tell us that Josh had swum a mile and a half and that he was hanging onto a dock when a couple heard him calling for help.

How did he survive all of that? And why did he try to take his life again? I feel nauseous again. And I can't stop crying. I am so sad for my son.

They move Josh from the ER to the surgery trauma intensive care unit (STICU). The surgical team says the fractures to his face need time to heal. He's not out of the woods yet, though. His eyesight needs to be monitored closely. His right lung is severely bruised, and the trauma to his muscles has resulted in copious amounts of lactic acid entering his bloodstream. The labs show elevated creatinine levels, which can indicate possible kidney failure. His creatinine level is fourteen when it should be one.

They run the lab work again.

While we're waiting for the second set of results, they will let us see Josh in the STICU. First, the doctor asks to meet with us in private. He explains that the trauma to Josh's entire muscular system could explain why his creatinine levels are so high—a result of his kidneys trying to expel the toxic lactic acid. Dangerously high levels could cause his kidneys to shut down. When the doctor reads the labs again, Josh's creatinine level is three.

Wow, his body is amazing. God is miraculous.

The doctor goes on to explain more about Josh's injuries and how he's amazed he survived.

I want to scream, *Yes, it's a miracle! God saved our son!*

They give Josh a sedative to help him sleep and begin to heal.

I hold his hand again.

Terrible thoughts run through my mind. *Josh could have drowned. I can't even imagine life without him.*

Aaron and I kiss Josh goodbye so he can rest. We walk outside and stand in the courtyard. Aaron lights a cigarette. I don't even remind him he should quit. We both voice our amazement about how our son survived.

"He is Superman!" Aaron tears up again. "We could've lost him tonight."

"Yes, I know." I look up at the stars. "It's a miracle."

I start sobbing. I feel such hopelessness. And hope at the same time.

We both agree that God saved our son's life. Josh had miraculously survived a 180-foot fall into the Charleston Harbor. He swam and floated a mile and a half to a dock near the USS *Yorktown*. He clung to the dock, moaning in pain. A young man with the same name heard him crying for help and pulled him out of the water and called 911.

God sent this amazing man who saved Josh's life. I will reach out to him to thank him.

We are silent again on the drive back home. I drop Aaron off at his place. I drive home with tears streaming down my face. The whole night is racing through my head.

How could my son be so depressed that he wanted to take his own life again?

"God, please help my son!" I yell out my window. I'm so mad, I have to pull over. I hit the steering wheel again and again and again until my hands hurt. I know it does not compare to the pain that my son is feeling.

It takes all of my courage and strength to drive home.

Once I'm safe at home, I sit in the driveway for a long time. I just cannot go in.

How long have I been out here? I must have dozed off.

I finally get out of the car and go inside.

Josh has been in the trauma unit for the past three weeks. I go to see him every day. I tell him I love him and hold his hand. I can see on his face that every inch of his body is in pain. He sleeps a lot. His eyesight is still blurry from the trauma. The swelling goes down a little each day. The bruises on his face change colors each day—black, purple, blue, yellow. His clavicle and cheekbones are still healing. The doctor says he should be able to see clearly again once the swelling dissipates completely.

My son's body is healing, but Josh remains flat and expressionless.

It breaks my heart to see my son so emotionally lifeless and his body so physically bruised. Every day, I pray for his emotional, mental, physical, and spiritual healing.

All the doctors and nurses are amazed that Josh survived the fall and that he doesn't have more injuries. Josh eats very little; the nurses continue to give him fluids with nutrients intravenously.

As I sit in a chair next to Josh's bed, I remind him that I am here for him. I tell him that his dad, his siblings, and his family love him. I write him a love letter. I put it in an uplifting card with a picture of Winnie-the-Pooh holding balloons on the front.

It remains unopened for days. *I am really sad that he didn't even open it.*

I have to cross that bridge every day to go to work and to see Josh. I scream at the top of my lungs every time I drive across it.

Why? Why does Josh have such severe depression? Why can't they help my son!

God, help my son! Please help my son!

When someone has a heart condition, we all understand the seriousness. Usually, there is something not working correctly with the chambers of the heart. Loved ones are very supportive and rally to find the best care. There are expert heart doctors and surgeons to help. Just as there may be malfunctions within the chambers of a person's heart, with depression there are malfunctions within the connections in a person's brain. When someone has a mental condition, however, no one truly understands. Very often, people think there is just something mentally not "right" with that person. But both patients need to be treated. And both patients need to be loved.

It infuriates me that there's a prejudice toward mental health and depression.

After Josh physically heals, they will move him to the MUSC Institute of Psychiatry. He's been there once before, as an adolescent, when he attempted to hang himself. Now he's an adult and will be in the adult unit. The staff promise to help him emotionally and mentally heal. They will monitor him and start electroconvulsive therapy (ECT) treatment.

Aaron's dad flies in to visit Josh. Josh breaks down when he sees his grandpa and is moved to tears. When I go to see him the next day, he cries with me too. I continue to tell him we all love him. I bring him gifts of a warm blanket, fresh clothes, and slippers. *I hope he will wear the clothes and slippers and use the blanket.*

A letter of thanks to the young man who saved my son.
Josh,

Words cannot begin to express my gratitude to you and your fiancée for saving our son. Your kindness and love are extraordinary. You were instrumental in saving his life. It's amazing to me that you both share the same first and middle name, Joshua Aaron.

To me you will always be an angel sent from God!

Blessings and love to you,

Maria

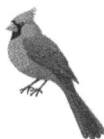

CHAPTER TWENTY-EIGHT

Space Between Recovery

Maria

Josh came home after a month in the hospital and the psychiatric unit. I have so many mixed feelings—I'm happy he's home, concerned about whether he's ready, and anxious about whether he will be safe. Josh is staying with his dad again. Aaron works from home, and we feel it's best that someone is always with Josh. Aaron and I know this is a big transition for him and a very big transition for us.

On my way to pick Josh up for his therapist appointment, so many thoughts are running through my mind.

I am trusting God. I am trusting God. I am trusting God.

So, to be transparent, I am freaking out inside. *I don't think my heart can handle Josh trying to hurt himself again. I know that God loves him so much. God has a purpose for his life. Josh is meant to be here, and I pray that he knows that.*

At Josh's therapist appointment, Dr. Allen asks me to join them for the first half of the session.

The doctor tells Josh that she's so happy he's alive. Then she asks the tough questions.

"Why did you jump?" she asks him.

Josh looks sad. "I didn't know what else to do."

"Can you share how you felt when you jumped?"

"Looking down, I was scared at first." Josh shudders. "Then the fear was gone."

"It really hurt when I hit the water," he goes on to explain. "I swam a little and then floated when I couldn't swim anymore. I didn't know if I could make it."

Josh pauses, and a tear runs down his cheek. "When I saw the dock, I started to swim faster. At that moment, I wanted to live."

I go to hug my son. I can't hold back my tears and my relief that he's alive.

Josh hugs me back.

"Josh, the young man who pulled you from the water has the same first and middle names as you," I share with him. "I sent him a letter to thank him." I wanted to tell him about this when his therapist was present.

I look at my son and can tell that he's touched.

"Maria, Josh is still having active suicidal thoughts since being in the hospital." Dr. Allen stops and looks at Josh. "He didn't tell me before he jumped, but we had a few phone conversations while he was still in the hospital."

"Oh, Josh." I reach over to touch his hand.

"I just feel so lonely. I didn't know how to tell you and Dad."

"Josh, please know that you can tell me or your dad anything, anytime!" I exclaim.

I step out of the room so Josh and the doctor can finish his session. In the waiting room, I pick up a magazine while I wait for him. He comes out about ten minutes later. He makes another appointment with the receptionist, and we head out to my car. Josh is quiet again during the car ride back to his dad's house.

"Josh, how are you feeling now?"

"I'm really tired, Mom."

I reach to touch his hand again to give him comfort. Honestly, I feel so futile in my efforts to help my son. I give him another hug when he gets out of the car to go into his dad's place.

Later, I call Aaron to share about Josh's therapist appointment. We both agree that we will continue to remind Josh that he can always come to us and tell us anything. When I get home, I order pizza for the three of us for dinner. I eat one slice and leave the rest for Audra and AJ.

I keep seeing Josh's bruised and battered face in the ER.

I'm so tired and tell the kids that I'm going to bed early. After brushing my teeth, I put on my pajamas and crawl into bed.

The silence is overwhelming. I start to hum "Amazing Grace." I pray that I will sleep tonight.

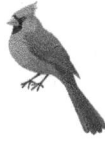

CHAPTER TWENTY-NINE

Small Steps Forward

Josh

Being at Dad's this time started out awful. We are moving into a bigger apartment in a few weeks. I didn't want to move at first. But this apartment is dark and depressing.

I realize I do want a change. So, I start packing up some of my things.

Dad's older cat, Snoops, has been acting weird the past few days. Right after Dad leaves to go get more boxes, she starts meowing and won't stop. I pick up my phone to call Dad, and Snoops has a seizure or something. I rush over to check on her.

"Dad, Snoops just had a seizure! She isn't moving!" I yell into the phone.

"I'm coming back!" Dad hangs up the phone.

I put my hand under Snoops's nose to feel if she is breathing. I know she is dead.

I start crying, seeing her lifeless body. Dad comes rushing through the front door.

He asks me if I want to help bury her. *No way*, I tell him.

Seeing the cat die really upset me. I've never witnessed anything die before.

Dad keeps asking me if I am OK. I tell him I am, because I really don't want to relive what happened.

Moving day comes, and we get everything moved to the new place. I like my new room a lot better. The whole place has a lot more light too. Daisy, the other cat, came with us, but she seems sad now. She misses her friend.

"Josh, I know it was hard to see Snoops die. Maybe we can get a new kitten."

"I will think about it, Dad."

To be honest, I know that Daisy would like a new little friend, and I would like it too. I spend the next few days getting my new room set up. The distraction is good for me. Our new place is surrounded by lots of trails. I grab my sneakers.

As I tie my laces, I yell to Dad, "I'm going out for a run!"

"Have fun!" Dad yells back from his bedroom.

I run a mile and get into a groove. It feels so good to just let the "high" of running wash over me. I decide to start running more.

Mom is coming over later to take me to my next appointment with Dr. Allen. I honestly don't want to go this time. Talking to her does help sometimes; I can clear my head by sharing the negative thoughts with her.

"Hey, Mom." I get into her car and put on my seat belt.

"Hi, it's great to see you." Mom smiles.

I love how Mom is always happy. Sometimes it wears off on me.

"You're much closer now. So, how do you like the new place?" she asks.

"I like it much better here," I tell her.

"Glad to hear that. Do you need anything for your room?"

"No, I'm all set."

"Well, Christmas is in a few months, so please let me know what you might want."

"OK, Mom. Let me think about it."

I really do need a laptop, but I always hate to ask for expensive things. I don't know why I feel that way. My parents are generous. They don't spoil us, but we always have what we need and more.

Mom waits in the waiting room while I go in to see Dr. Allen. I decide to tell the doctor about Snoops.

"I didn't want to talk about seeing the cat die, because it's like it's happening again."

"Josh, talking about it can bring up the emotions you felt seeing Snoops die. What did you feel then, and what do you feel now?"

"I was scared then, and now I'm really sad. Dad offered to get a new kitten."

"How do you feel about getting a new cat?" Dr. Allen asks me.

"I don't want one just to replace Snoops. But I think that Daisy, our other cat, would really like a friend."

"Think about your dad's offer," Dr. Allen encourages me.

"I will." I do think I would like a new kitten. "Also, I have had fewer suicidal thoughts."

"Josh, I'm so happy to hear that." Dr. Allen pauses. "I would like you to consider ways you can enjoy life again. Getting a new cat and building that connection can be a precursor to building new relationships."

I nod and then look down. Hanging out with a new kitten will be a lot easier than hanging out with my old friends.

We schedule my next appointment, and the doctor updates my medicine.

"How did it go?" Mom asks when we are back in the car.

"It went well. I did talk about Snoops."

"It must have been very upsetting to witness that."

"Yeah, it was. Dad suggested getting a new kitten."

"What do you think?" Mom questions.

"At first, I didn't want a kitten. Now I think that it would be a good thing."

Mom smiles. "You want to go get some lunch?"

"Yes, I'm starving." We go to a restaurant near Dad's place. Mom gets a salad, and I get their famous burger and fries.

"Mom, do you think I could get a new laptop for Christmas? I could use a new one."

"Yes, pick out the one you want." Mom seems happy to have a gift idea for me.

We finish our lunch and head back to her car.

"We should do lunch more often," Mom suggests as we are driving back.

"Yeah, thanks for lunch today." I smile as I get out of the car.

"You're so welcome," Mom responds.

I feel lighter when I walk through the front door.

"Hey, Dad, I'm home," I shout, wondering where he is.

"Hi, I'm out here on the porch. How was your appointment?"

"It was really good. I did talk about Snoops."

"Oh, yeah?" Dad looks up.

"Yes, and I would like a new kitten for Christmas," I share with a big smile.

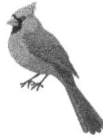

CHAPTER THIRTY

New Horizons

Maria

Audra was accepted to the University of Rhode Island. Grant is driving the fourteen hours with us to take her to college. He and I agreed it would be good for both of them to spend some quality time together. Audra has told me she really likes Grant. I'm really excited about the trip. After we get my daughter moved in, Grant and I are going to spend a week in New York City. Grant has never been, and I'm excited to explore the city together.

We head out the Saturday before Labor Day. Grant drives most of the trip, but Audra and I take over driving once or twice. I forgot how monotonous it is driving North on I-95. It's beautiful to see more hills and just a touch of color on the trees the farther North we go. We listen to several comedians on SiriusXM, along with some rock, country, and pop music. We talk about Audra's new school. She will be studying marine biology. Her college is tucked within the quaint town of Kingston, Rhode Island. After fourteen hours, we turn right onto the tree-lined drive showcasing the historic homes where the professors live. We continue down the drive toward the dorms. We pull up in front of Audra's dorm, and she hops out to check in.

"My room is on the second floor," she lets us know when she gets back in the car.

"OK, let's start unloading your stuff." Grant is a natural leader.

I get teary when everything is unloaded in Audra's dorm room. Her roommate moved in earlier. I help Audra get her bed made and her desk organized. We decorate the wall next to her bed with string lights and pictures of family and friends. Grant gives Audra a hug and a few words of wisdom. Then he leaves to wait for me outside.

"Mom, thank you so much for all your help." Audra comes over to hug me.

"You're so welcome." I hug her tight.

"Remember, Nana is only two hours from here," Audra reminds me.

"I know, and that makes me feel better, knowing you have family close." I wink at her.

"I love you, Mom."

"I love you too. Goodbye, sweetheart." I hug her once more and head downstairs to meet Grant. He gives me a big hug, and I let my tears fall.

"You OK, sweetheart?" Grant looks into my eyes.

"I will be." I wipe my tears with my sleeve.

"You ready to go to New York City?" he asks.

"I am. Let's go." We walk hand in hand to the car.

Four hours later, we are entering the Big Apple. Grant's whole demeanor changes as he navigates among the hectic, horn-honking cars, trucks, and buses. I keep reminding him this is just the beginning of the hustle of the big city. We drop off our suitcases at the hotel. Grant and I quickly return the car we rented for the trip. We will be flying home.

Back in our hotel room, we get dressed up for our first evening in New York City. Grant made reservations for dinner at Carmine's. After dinner, we are going to see a Broadway musical, a surprise for me.

We take a cab to the restaurant. The hostess leads us to our table—it's lit by an ivory candle in a crystal votive that sends sparkling stars all over the table. Grant orders a bottle of pinot noir, and we place our orders. Grant has the chicken parmigiana, and I opt for the shrimp fra diavolo. We share our food, and both meals are delicious. After dinner, we head across the street to see *The Phantom of the Opera*. I have seen many Broadway musicals, but I have not had the opportunity to see this show. I love every minute of it.

"Thank you so much. I had a wonderful evening." I turn to Grant and kiss him.

"You're welcome." He kisses me back.

We walk back to the hotel hand in hand. I feel so much love for Grant. I know he is the man meant for me.

We are up early the next morning. Grant is making coffee for me and tea for himself. We have to be at the Megyn Kelly Show by eight o'clock to get checked in. Luckily, we can walk there, and we even have a few minutes to spare.

The show is a lot of fun, and Grant even knows one of the security guards. *It really is a small world.* Next on the agenda is Tiffany's. The clasp on my bracelet needs to be fixed.

I look at Grant, and he seems flustered. He keeps insisting that we do Tiffany's tomorrow. But we're close to the store, and we still have plenty of time to make our lunch reservation at the Central Park Boathouse.

"I am all set. They can repair my bracelet today, and we can come back to get it tomorrow," I relay to Grant as I meet him in the waiting area.

"We really have to hurry if we are going to make our lunch reservation," he insists.

"Can you call and see if they have a later time available?" I ask.

"I guess I can." Grant pulls out his phone. "Although I made this reservation three months ago."

Grant calls the Boathouse, and luckily, they are able to move our reservation to one o'clock this afternoon. So, we take a taxi back to the hotel to change since it's ninety-five degrees out. We are going to bike in Central Park.

After walking from the hotel to the bike rental shop, we are given our bikes. The shop is just across the street from the park, so we walk our bikes to the park entrance.

I'm able to coast the first half mile since the path is downhill. However, as the path levels out and I start to pedal, I realize there's something wrong with my bike. The wheels are moving, but there's a lot of friction.

"Grant, I can't seem to pedal this bike."

"What's wrong with it?" he asks with a little more frustration.

"It seems like it's catching on something when I try to pedal."

"Well, we're almost there, and it's downhill from here."

So I coast the rest of the way and try not to pedal at all. We arrive at the Boathouse at 12:30.

"Guess we made our original reservation." Grant winks at me. "Let's walk our bikes up to Bethesda Fountain to wait."

"Honey, I'm really hot. But OK." I follow him toward the fountain.

I park my bike next to the lake to try to get a breeze.

"Sweetheart, let's get a picture by the fountain," Grant suggests.

"Someone may take our bikes," I respond.

Grant insists, so I follow him to the fountain and sit on the edge. He goes in search of someone to take our picture.

I look down and see that my shoelace is undone. Once I have tied my shoe and look up, Grant is in front of me; he's on one knee.

"Maria, I'm the luckiest man to have met you. I love you. Will you marry me?"

"Yes!" I am overwhelmed with emotion and love for him. He helps me stand up and kisses me.

A very nice French couple recorded our proposal. They congratulate us and return Grant's phone. Grant pulls me into a hug and kisses me passionately.

"Maria, I love you so much!" He keeps kissing me.

"I love you and can't wait to be your wife." I feel such joy.

We walk our bikes back to the restaurant and lock them in the bike rack. Grant chuckles as he notices my chain is hanging off my bike.

"Welcome to the Boathouse. Right this way." The hostess leads us to our seats after Grant gives his last name. In time, that will be my last name too.

"Hi, my name is Howard, and I will be your server." The waiter comes to our table as we sit down. "May I get each of you a drink to start?"

"Champagne, please," Grant responds, smiling at me. "We just got engaged."

"Congratulations! Allow me to go and get a bottle we reserve for special occasions."

"Thank you," we both say at the same time.

The waiter returns with a bottle of champagne and two champagne flutes. He opens the bottle and pours each of us a glass.

"To my beautiful bride-to-be. I love you."

"To my handsome husband-to-be. I love you."

We clink our glasses together. Both of us are so excited; we talk nonstop about the wedding and the honeymoon.

But more importantly, we talk about our new life together.

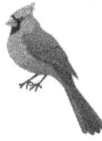

CHAPTER THIRTY-ONE

Time to Live

Josh

This fall, I have more and more moments when I feel good. I don't know if it's the ECT treatments that have helped or the new depression medication. I am even sleeping better.

If I'm meant to be here, I want to get my life on track. One thing I can control is my physical health. I've been running again. It's the best exercise for me. I get that natural high from running that always helps me feel better. I feel so energized and don't have to battle the headaches that I sometimes get after smoking pot.

I also get exercise refereeing soccer games for the little kids. It's not a career path for me, but it gives me some spending cash.

And Dad and I are spending more time together. We both like to eat well. Last night, we grilled steaks together and made baked potatoes and a spinach salad. After dinner, we watched the NC State football game against the University of North Carolina.

"Hey, Dad, you still going downtown to the market today?" I ask when I walk into the living room. It makes me happy thinking about buying Christmas gifts.

"Yeah, would you like to come with me?" Dad asks as he shuts his computer down.

"Yeah, I want to find Christmas gifts for Mom, AJ, Audra, and Curt."

"We can leave in five minutes." Dad goes into his room to get his keys and shoes.

I know that spending time with my family and friends helps me feel better. But it's been a year since I have seen many of my friends. *They know about my depression and my suicide attempts. Will they really want to spend time with me?*

I will reach out to Alec when he is home from college over Christmas.

His friendship is really important to me. I hope we can still be good friends.

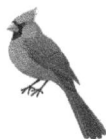

CHAPTER THIRTY-TWO

Seasonal Emotions

Maria

Christmas is here again. Audra will be home from college in a week. I miss her so much. I will call her later to get some gift ideas. I have to finish shopping and decorate the rest of the house too. I'm trying to get into the Christmas spirit, but this year I'm really struggling, and I feel like Scrooge.

I put the radio on, playing a Christmas station while I start to make my coffee.

"Mom, what's for breakfast?" AJ asks, coming into the kitchen.

"Would you like pancakes this morning?" I ask him.

"Oh yes, let me know when they're ready." He returns to his room with a glass of orange juice.

I pull out the oil and add water to the pancake mix. I even add chocolate chips to the batter. AJ comes back downstairs ten minutes later, as soon as he smells them cooking.

"Thanks, Mom."

"You're so welcome. I know how much you like chocolate-chip pancakes."

AJ eats four pancakes and drinks another glass of orange juice. I smile at my growing boy, who's taller than me now.

"I'm going to take a shower and head over to Lance's house."

"OK, have fun," I respond.

I clean up the kitchen and take my coffee cup out on the back porch.

I still feel fear from time to time, thinking about Josh. I honestly think I may have post-traumatic stress syndrome. In college, I talked to a psychiatrist about my parents' divorce, and Aaron and I went to a few sessions together during our separation. It helped a little to talk about our marriage struggles.

I give Josh credit—it's not easy to talk to someone about your feelings and the struggles going on in your life.

I open my iPad and look for local therapists. Maybe Dr. Allen could give me some recommendations.

Just then, the phone rings.

"Hi, Grant, how are you?" I answer the phone.

"I'm good. I miss you. Whatcha doing today?" he asks me.

"I'm on my back porch, contemplating decorating the house. How about you?"

"Christmas shopping. Would you like to go to a Christmas concert with me on Friday night?" Grant asks enthusiastically. "I can pick you up that evening at six o'clock."

"Ah, shopping, I have to do that too. Yes, I would love to go to a Christmas concert with you." Maybe that will help me get in the Christmas spirit.

"Perfect, I can't wait to see you on Friday!"

Hanging up the phone, I'm still smiling. Grant always makes me feel better. Now I'm motivated to decorate, and I pull out all the Christmas decorations. I even put on my favorite Christmas CD.

"Have Yourself a Merry Little Christmas" is playing, and I feel a little less like Scrooge. I finish decorating downstairs and decide that's enough for today. A hot bubble bath sounds good to me. I head upstairs to start running the water and find my favorite bubble bath. *Is it too early in the day to have a glass of wine?*

I decide it's too early. Once in the tub, I let the hot water melt away the tension.

Why am I letting Christmas bother me this year? Christmas always brings me joy. I close my eyes and just let music lull me to another world. Several songs later, I realize it's my fear that is getting in the way of my joy again. *I will not let fear rob me of my joy or make me crazy.* I let the water drain and wrap myself in the biggest, fluffiest towel. I dress in my favorite red sweater and jeans. I feel festive and hopeful for a merry Christmas.

I pick up the phone to call Audra. "Hi, Audra, I'm heading to the mall. Any thoughts on gifts for you and your brothers?"

"Mom, Christmas is in two weeks," she reminds me.

"Yes, I know, I'm a bit behind."

"I can text you a few suggestions," she offers.

"Audra, anything you want to do for Christmas?" I ask her.

"Can we go to The Charleston Place hotel when they have snow and hot chocolate?"

"Yes, I love that!" I am happy to make Christmas memories with her.

"I will also text you my flight information," Audra adds.

"Thank you. Can't wait to see you on Friday. Love you," I say, all in one breath.

I grab my purse and sunglasses and head out the front door. I can find a few last-minute things at the mall for the kids. I park at the mall and head into Barnes & Noble first. I find myself in the self-help section. There are several books on post-traumatic stress on the shelf. I read several paragraphs in a few books. I chicken out and don't purchase any of them because I first want to get guidance from a therapist. I will call one of the local therapists on Monday.

I don't want to feel the sadness about Josh that creeps in more and more.

Walking around aimlessly for twenty minutes, I finally go into the department store. I find pajamas for each of the kids. One of my favorite traditions is buying them matching pajamas for Christmas. The kids open them on Christmas Eve and sleep in their new pajamas. Even as teenagers, they still enjoy this tradition. I'm happy to have gotten something else done for Christmas.

Somewhat inspired, I decide to go to the grocery store to get ingredients to make Christmas cookies. The grocery store is packed. I manage to find all the ingredients for the kids' favorite Christmas cookies—gingerbread for Curt, chocolate crinkles for Josh, Italian cookies for Audra, and Christmas-cutout sugar cookies for AJ. I also get a pot roast, potatoes, and carrots for dinner. As I head to the front of the store to check out, I run right into Janet, Alec's mom.

"Hi, how are you?" she practically shouts at me.

"Hi, been hanging in there. How are you?" I quietly mumble.

"Alec comes home this week for Christmas. I'm just picking up some of his favorites."

"Audra comes home this week too," I say, hoping she will not ask about Josh in the grocery store.

"How is Josh?" she asks next.

"He's doing better," I manage to say without crying.

"Maybe the boys could see each other over the holidays."

"Yeah, that might work. Great to see you. Merry Christmas," I say quickly and hurry off before I start bawling in the store. Thank goodness for self-checkout.

I drive straight home and unload the groceries. I prepare the pot roast in the crockpot and turn it on. Pulling out the family cookbook, I start making the dough for the gingerbread and the Christmas sugar cookies. The phone rings, and Aaron starts talking as soon as I say hello.

"I'm going out of town to see my parents over the holidays. Can Josh stay with you the week after Christmas?"

"Yes, he can, and I can take him to his therapist appointment too. And, Aaron, I'm going to reach out to a therapist and make an appointment for me. You may want to see someone too."

"Maria, you know I hate talking about my feelings."

"Yes, I know." I bite my lip so as not to say anything else.

I say goodbye and hang up the phone. Focusing my attention back on making the cookies, I feel my body relax. Cooking, bubble baths, the beach, and gardening are my escapes.

AJ comes home just as I pull the first batch of cookies from the oven.

"Do I smell cookies?" He walks right into the kitchen.

"Yes, I made your favorite—Christmas sugar cookies."

"May I have some?" AJ asks with a huge grin on his face.

"You want to help me decorate the cookies?" I ask.

"Yes. Can I eat some as we decorate?"

"Of course. Wash your hands first." He does what I ask. Picking up a cookie, he takes a bite. "Thanks, Mom. These are great."

"You're welcome." We decorate Santa Clauses, candy canes, and more. We both sing along to the Christmas carols playing in the background. AJ loves Christmas music, just like me.

It makes me happy when my kids are happy.

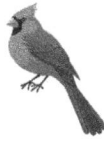

CHAPTER THIRTY-THREE

Gifts of Presence

Josh

Christmas was yesterday, and Mom always makes it great. I did get a new laptop from her. Dad got me a new kitten; I named her Emily. She follows me everywhere and sleeps with me too. I really like having her around. Dad's going to visit his parents until New Year's Day. I didn't want to go. I love my grandparents, but I don't want to talk about my feelings or explain what's been happening. So, I'm going to stay with Mom. It will be good to spend more time with her and my siblings. The frustrating thing is that my parents don't trust me to stay alone. I'm doing better, but I don't have the best track record.

Mom said she invited Alec and his mom over for dinner one night. It will be great and weird at the same time to see him. I have not talked to him since I left college. *I still consider him my best friend. I hope that he does too, but I'm not sure that he does.*

"Hey, Dad, do you know where my green sweater is?" I question Dad.

"It's folded on top of the dryer in the laundry room," Dad responds.

"Thanks." I head to the laundry room.

"You almost done packing?" Dad asks when I walk back into the kitchen.

"Yeah, almost," I tell him.

"I put the new cat food on the shelf in the pantry," Dad continues.

"I will come by three or four times to feed them."

"OK, I will finish packing, and then we can both go." Dad heads to his room.

I put my favorite sweaters, a few Hawaiian shirts, and some khakis, underwear, and socks in my duffel bag. I never know what the weather will be like in Charleston this time of year. I can always grab another shirt or sweater when I come back to feed the cats.

"I'm ready, Dad."

"OK, let's go." Dad checks the apartment one more time.

We both head down in the elevator.

"I love you, Josh," Dad says as he comes over to hug me.

"I love you too, Dad." We haven't hugged like that in a while.

I feel closer to Dad. I realize that me living with him has been good for both of us.

"See you in a week." Dad turns toward his car.

"Bye, Dad. Have a safe trip." I jump in my car.

I blast my music, this time to enjoy it and not just to drown out my thoughts.

"Hi, Josh. We are all in the living room," Mom announces when I close the front door.

"Hi, what's everyone doing?" I ask.

"Watching *Christmas Vacation*, even though Christmas is over," AJ chimes in.

"Great movie." I find a seat with my family.

I'm happy to be here with them, but I'm far away in my thoughts.

"So, Alec and his mom are coming over to dinner tomorrow night," Mom says when the movie is over.

"Oh, OK." I'm not sure how excited Alec will be about coming over to see me.

"I can make fried chicken, mashed potatoes, and green beans," Mom continues.

She used to make fried chicken for Alec and me all the time. I'm thankful Mom remembers how much we both love it.

"Thanks, Mom. I'm going to take my stuff up to my room."

"We are just having pizza tonight. I will order it in a little while."

Sitting on my bed, I start having the same sad thoughts.

"Enough!" I say out loud. I will see my friends and go to school and get back to being me.

I head back downstairs. "Mom, thank you for inviting Alec. I'm looking forward to seeing him."

"You're welcome." Mom smiles.

"I want to ask you if your offer to take me to the Amen Clinic is still good?" I ask her.

"Yes, of course. I can call next week to schedule an appointment."

"Thank you, Mom. I want to start feeling better." I smile at her.

I feel hopeful. *I want to find out why I have been so depressed for so long.*

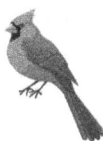

CHAPTER THIRTY-FOUR
The Amen Clinic

Maria

Josh asked me to take him to the Amen Clinic over the holidays. In the fall, I shared with him that the clinic did brain SPECT imaging. They would be able to give him insight into his depression and addiction. It was not until after Christmas that he finally agreed; I think he has been afraid to discover what is wrong.

I'm nervous while driving to pick Josh up from his dad's house. *I really hope the Amen Clinic can provide answers about his depression.* The minute Josh gets in the car, I start to relax. We talk, laugh, and listen to music. Josh is very passionate about sharing his new age music with me.

I don't know why I was nervous; we're having a great road trip together.

Stopping only once for breakfast, we make it to Atlanta in five hours. We check into the hotel and start planning where to have an early dinner. Right across the street is a Japanese restaurant. We both agree that's perfect.

At dinner, Josh is quiet again.

"Are you nervous or excited or both about tomorrow?" I finally ask him.

"I'm ready to figure out why I've been feeling this way." Josh rubs his hands together.

I wonder what the tests will show us. I really hope they can help Josh. We finish our chicken and steak hibachi, and I pay the check.

Later, in our room, we watch *Friends* on TV. After watching Monica and Chandler's rehearsal dinner episode, we're both ready to turn in for the night.

In the morning, we head to the clinic bright and early. There is an older couple, and a young girl, maybe ten years old, with her mom. The staff call Josh back. I pass several hours in the waiting room reading *People* magazines. When Josh's tests are done, it's lunchtime. It's raining outside, and I forgot my umbrella. We run across the street and take cover in the parking garage. We head to a local mall to get lunch and walk around. Later that afternoon, we go back to the hotel to rest and freshen up. Josh will have more tests tomorrow morning.

"Josh, would you like to see more of Atlanta?"

"Sure, Mom."

So, Josh and I head to the other side of town. The rain has stopped, and we drive to a cute neighborhood with shops and restaurants. Josh is patient while I browse through a boutique with local art. We stumble upon a fun, eclectic restaurant for dinner.

I'm so happy spending time with my son.

"Mom, thank you again for this trip to Atlanta and for paying for the tests at the Amen Clinic."

"You're so welcome. I know how important it is for you to find out why you have been depressed." *I want to give Josh hope they will be able to offer him a solution.*

Back at the hotel, we watch the next episode of *Friends*—Monica and Chandler's wedding day. We set several alarms to get up early the next day and head to bed.

Waking up the next morning, I have a strange feeling of worry. *Maria, they will be able to give Josh an answer*, I tell myself.

Back at the clinic, Josh looks excited. They call his name, and he smiles at me as he goes through the patient door. I sigh in relief. After two days of brain scans and a lot of waiting, Josh and I meet with Dr. Brennan right before noon. The doctor explains that Josh's concussion did affect the area of the brain that influences addictive tendencies and can cause depression and suicidal thoughts. I look at Josh, and he nods back.

Wow, the concussions did affect Josh's brain negatively.

The doctor explains several positive ways to heal Josh's brain, including taking omega-3 and other supplements. Often, he tells us, medications just treat the symptoms and don't heal the affected area of the brain. Dr. Brennan goes on to discuss other alternatives, including hallucinogenic LSD therapies.

I don't think that would be best for Josh right now. However, Josh is curious to hear more about the hallucinogenic therapies. The doctor explains they are conducted in a controlled environment.

Josh agrees to start taking some of the recommended supplements. I thank the doctor for his time.

Checking out at the clinic desk, I purchase two bottles of supplements for Josh. As we are leaving the building, I turn to him. "I thought the doctor's explanation and all we learned today was really helpful."

"It was OK," Josh responds flatly.

We walk to the parking garage so we can head home.

As we get into the car, Josh insists he has been doing the best thing for himself by taking hallucinogens.

"Dr. Brennan did explain some about the new hallucinogenic therapy, but, Josh, taking them by yourself is dangerous," I try to explain to him.

I wish that the doctor had never mentioned that type of therapy.

"My therapist has shared about hallucinogenic therapy," Josh turns to me to say. "Mom, stop being unintelligent and narrow-minded."

I'm quite upset that he voiced that to me. I feel tears welling up in my eyes.

"Josh, I would like you to try the healthy alternatives that Dr. Brennan suggested to heal your brain."

Josh gets more agitated that the doctor couldn't explain the recent pressure in the back of his head. I tell him that the doctor explained the best he could and that Josh can read his notes. Josh continues to get more upset with me; he stops talking altogether. I decide it's best to stop, get some air, and find something to eat. When I pull into the parking lot of the restaurant, Josh gets out of the car. He goes to the trunk to get his bag and then walks away.

"Don't follow me!" he yells.

I can't breathe as fear grips me.

I call Aaron to tell him what is happening. "Josh is very upset after our conversation about the doctor's recommendations. When I stopped the car to get lunch, he got his bag and took off!"

"I will call and talk to him." Aaron hangs up.

When Aaron calls me back, he said Josh told him he will take the bus home.

What do I do? With tears streaming down my face, I call Grant.

"Josh walked away after we stopped for something to eat on our way home. I'm so worried about him," I say.

"Wow, that must have really upset you," Grant responds. And all of sudden, I'm flooded with so many emotions.

"I'm really scared," I share with him. "But I'm furious that Josh walked away from me after all I have done for him!"

"Maria, you have every right to be angry. Why don't you stay another night? Maybe Josh will come back to the hotel," Grant offers. "I will pay for the additional night."

"Grant, I can't ask you to do that."

"Maria, I'm offering."

"Thank you! I'm too upset to drive." I accept his offer.

"Honey, he will be OK," Grant says to make me feel better.

"Thank you. I love you. I will call you in the morning." I hang up the phone and get into the car to head to the hotel. My hands are shaking and feel cold and clammy.

Josh doesn't call or come to the hotel. I'm terrified that he won't come back home or that he will be seriously hurt.

What if he tries to take his life again? I cry myself to sleep.

I wake up at six o'clock the next morning and check the bus schedule online. There are two buses from Atlanta to Charleston. By bus, the journey will take eight hours; I pray Josh will take one home.

I find the coffee maker and make my first cup of coffee. Just then, the phone rings.

"Hi, have you heard from him?" Aaron asks.

"No, I haven't. Did he text or email your family?" I ask hopefully.

"No one has heard from him. I hope he got on a bus back to Charleston," Aaron adds.

"Me too. Please let me know if you hear something." I hang up.

I call Grant to let him know that Josh didn't come back and I'm coming home. I check out of the hotel and begin the five-hour drive back to Charleston. I cry most of the drive. When I get home, I am emotionally, mentally, and physically exhausted.

I just want to hear that Josh made it safely home. Right before dinner, the phone rings.

"Maria, Josh came back twenty minutes ago. He took the early bus back and walked five miles from downtown Charleston to Daniel Island." Aaron is very upset. "We had a fight."

"What did you fight about?" I question him.

"He said that I haven't been a good dad and he's moving out."

"Oh, I'm so sorry. You're a great dad!" I hope Aaron knows that. "What do we do?"

"I don't know. We can talk later." Aaron hangs up.

I'm angry, fearful, sad, and discouraged.

Feeling exhausted, I head to bed. As I'm about to turn off the bedside lamp, I see my Bible. I open it to Proverbs and to one of my favorite verses, Proverbs 3:5–6: *Trust in the Lord with all your heart, and do not lean on your own understanding. In all your ways acknowledge Him, and He will direct your paths.*

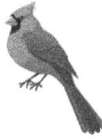

CHAPTER THIRTY-FIVE

Invisible Battles

I walk this empty street ...
Where the city sleeps
And I'm the only one ...
My shadow's the only one that walks beside me ...
Sometimes, I wish someone out there will find me
—"Boulevard of Broken Dreams," Green Day

Josh

Listening to the doctor tell me about my brain is so surreal. He explains that the concussion did impact the area of my brain that affects addiction and depression. Deep down, I already knew that. He shares about hallucinogenic therapy. I've done that on my own already. Yeah, I know it may not have been the best way; however, I know how much I'm taking.

Mom starts asking lots of questions. *Why doesn't she trust that I know what helps me?*

I'm ready to go when the doctor talks about healing my brain with supplements. Mom hears him say "healthy ways" to heal my brain, and we're here for another ten minutes.

Mom bought some supplements; I know that I won't take them. I've been dealing with depression for six years. Hallucinogens are really the only thing that makes me feel better, and if that's something they're using in therapy, that's good enough for me.

The doctor could not even explain the pressure I feel at the back of my head. I've recently been having a dull pain in my head, which I shared with Dr. Allen at my last visit. This doctor asked me if I had any pain, and I said the pain is worse when I wake up. I hoped he might explain it or provide a solution to make it go away.

But once again, even doctors don't really know how to explain the emotional or physical symptoms of depression. I try to explain how I feel, but no one can really help me.

As we get in the car, Mom does not stop talking about the supplements.

Now I'm getting mad. *Just stop talking, Mom.*

Finally, she stops talking, noticing my silence. She gets off the highway and pulls up to a restaurant. I don't want food, and I don't want to be around her anymore.

I get out and get my bag, and I walk away.

Why is she following me? I'm not going back to Charleston with her. Who is she talking to on the phone?

Dad calls to ask me to go back with Mom. I hang up on Dad and turn off my phone. I walk for half an hour. When I turn my phone back on, there are twenty or so messages. I delete them all. While walking, I decide to take the bus back to Charleston. I google the closest bus depot, and it's five miles away. I have some money, but not enough.

I text Matt, even though I have not talked to him since I left Clemson. He says he can send me some money for the bus via Venmo. It will take me forty-five minutes to get to the bus station. I want to get there before dark. I see a McDonald's on the way. I get a Happy Meal. I look at the paper wrapper on the burger, feeling far from happy. I shove the food in my mouth while I'm walking.

Walking does clear my mind a little.

I make it to the train station by seven o'clock, just before sunset.

Thank goodness for daylight savings last week.

Now I have to wait for the first bus in the morning.

Luckily, I have my phone charger. I plug it in the wall behind the row of seats by the window. I sit down, put in my earbuds, and choose my favorite Spotify station.

I will stay awake tonight and sleep on the bus.

It's going to be a long night.

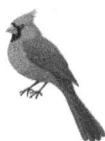

CHAPTER THIRTY-SIX

True Uncertainty

Maria

I have not heard from Josh since he walked away from me and took the bus home from Atlanta to Charleston. Almost two weeks later, he sends me a text.

Hi, Mom, I'm in Atlantic City.

Are you OK? What are you doing there? I reply.

I've been talking to Dad's sister, Aunt Rachel. At Christmas, Dad offered to take me to Las Vegas for my birthday. Well, now I'm not going to Vegas with Dad since he no longer wants to take me. Aunt Rachel suggested Atlantic City. I took the bus from Charleston. Just got here.

Oh, wow, I text back, feeling the worry rise in me once again.

As if he knows that, Josh writes, *I'm good, Mom. I was with friends in Charleston.*

Oh, I text back.

I'm sorry, Mom. Reading Josh's text, anger rushes back in.

I breathe in and out. I know Josh is truly sorry. I will forgive him.

Josh, I forgive you. I'm sorry, I just wanted you to understand the damage to your brain.

Mom, I understand. I forgive you. I know I have to start healing my brain, he texts back.

So, what are you going to do first in Atlantic City? I ask tentatively.

Gamble, Mom, what else? he writes back. *I have some money.*

I can send you $100, even though you know I really don't like gambling.

I know, but I'm here to gamble. Thank you, Mom.

You're welcome, good night. I will see how you did in the morning. Love you.

Love you too, Mom. Night.

I couldn't sleep at all last night. I send Josh a text to encourage him to use the money to get a hotel, knowing he would just stay up. I also sent a message to his dad, telling him that Josh is in Atlantic City. I'm distracted all day at work, wondering if Josh is OK.

Finally, that afternoon I send him a text.

Hi, how's it going? I ask.

Great, Mom, he immediately writes back. I feel my whole body relax.

Just been playing poker. I'm up and down, he continues.

Oh, sounds fun, I text. Right then, I decide to pay for a hotel for him for two nights.

Hey, I bet you are tired. I'm going to pay for Bally's Hotel for two nights.

You don't have to do that, Mom, he responds.

I know. I want to give this to you.

Thanks, Mom.

I book a room for him for two nights. Josh goes right to the hotel to check in.

Mom, thanks again. I'm going to get some sleep.

You're welcome. Sleep well. I love you.

Love you too, Mom.

I feel some relief, but what's he going to do after those two nights? In response to my question, Aaron sends me a text at that moment.

My sister is driving down from Massachusetts to stay with Josh for a few nights in Atlantic City.

I have always loved how much she cares about her niece and nephews, especially Josh, I text back to him.

After another terrible night's sleep, I'm running late for work. Just then, my mom calls.

"Hi, Mom, I'm doing all right. How are you?" I ask as I get into my car, putting the key in the ignition.

"I'm good, but the weather has been rainy here in Arizona." Mom moved to Arizona fifteen years ago.

"Josh is taking a bus from Atlantic City to visit me," Mom continues.

"Oh, I know you will be happy to see him. When is he taking a bus there?"

"I'm glad he wants to spend some time with me. He will take the first bus on Friday from Atlantic City to Nashville. And then take the second bus from Nashville to Phoenix."

"Mom, I know you know all that Josh has been through."

"Yes, and I hope spending time with his family will help him." Mom lets out a sigh.

"Please let me know when he gets to Arizona," I remind her.

"I will let you know. Love you, Maria."

"I love you too, Mom."

I hang up the phone with another sigh of relief. *God is really watching over my son.*

When I get to work, I send a text to Josh to ask him what his plans are. He responds back right away.

Yes, Mom. I'm taking a bus to Arizona to see Mom-mom.

When do you leave? I text again.

This Friday, he replies.

Enjoy the next few days in Atlantic City with your aunt.

I will. Thanks, Mom.

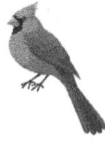

CHAPTER THIRTY-SEVEN

Heading West

Josh

I'm on another bus, this time heading out West. I was not in a very good state of mind when I took the bus home from Atlanta. I was angry and had so much "crazy" energy. That's the only way I can explain it. Then the sadness crept in and suffocated me. No matter how much Mom and Dad help me, it's frustrating being given their opinions constantly. I don't even know my own voice. This time I'm choosing to go to Arizona to see my grandmother.

I slept a lot of the trip, but I do appreciate the change of scenery. For the past two hours, the terrain has been golden desert and red rock mountains. Such a stark contrast to the green marshes and blue ocean.

"Phoenix, next stop," the bus driver announces to all of us on the bus. I put my travel pillow and headphones in my backpack.

Mom-mom is picking me up at the bus stop. I see her as I get off the bus.

"Hi, Josh, it's so great to see you," she says as she approaches me.

"You too," I say, giving her a big hug.

"I bet you're hungry." I nod. She continues, "There's a great burger place not far from here."

We head to the restaurant, and we're seated right away. Mom-mom asks me question after question about the Atlanta trip, my trip to Atlantic City, and my bus ride out to see her. She's so excited for me to be here and shares her plans for my stay.

I answer all her questions, but she finally realizes how tired I am.

"Let's get the check and head home so you can turn in early tonight."

I'm grateful she's so intuitive and for this time with her to decide my next steps.

We cover a lot of the state of Arizona in three weeks—we visit Sedona, Scottsdale, and even the Grand Canyon.

I remember coming out with Mom and Dad and my siblings to see the Grand Canyon when I was younger. We took a funny family picture as Curt pretended he was hanging over the edge. As an adult, I now appreciate the beauty and grandeur of the Grand Canyon.

Between our trips around the state, Mom-mom and I play card games. I win poker every time. It's great just to relax and go with the flow. I also spend time on the computer, researching colleges in California. Aunt Rachel helps me find a great tech school in San Francisco. She's helping me to persuade Mom and Dad that it's a good school for me.

I believe this opportunity to be on my own is the right thing for me. *But will being on the other side of the country be?*

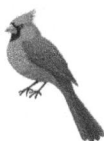

CHAPTER THIRTY-EIGHT

Distant Connection

Maria

After visiting my mom, Josh took another bus to San Francisco. He enrolled in a two-year computer program and got financing all on his own.

I understand Josh wants to be on his own. I'm proud of him, but I'm afraid too.

The first month, we spoke several times and texted most days. He says he's enjoying his classes and sleeping better.

To be honest, I feel he avoided the hard conversations—by walking away from me in Atlanta and fighting with his dad and moving out—and the real reason he ran away to the other side of the country. *I know Josh has always had trouble sharing his emotions. I really need a break from constantly worrying if he will be OK.*

Grant and I are about to leave for a cruise in the Caribbean. Our wedding is on New Year's Eve, and we will only have one night for a honeymoon, so we decided to have a pre-wedding honeymoon. I ask

Aaron to be in contact with Josh while we're gone. Aaron and I really do have a friendly relationship now.

Grant and I are flying to Miami, and then we will leave from the port there.

I'm so ready for a vacation.

Several days out at sea have relaxed me. We're having so much fun. One night at dinner, Josh sends me a text.

Mom, I'm not doing well. I'm feeling really depressed again. I don't know what to do.

My heart sinks. I'm thousands of miles away from him. I quickly excuse myself from the table as tears well up in my eyes. I walk to the top deck and call Josh.

"Mom," he responds on the third ring.

"Hi, I just got your text." I exhale, relieved to hear his voice.

"Mom, I'm still very sad. Will I ever feel better?" Josh chokes up.

"I'm so sorry, Josh. Are you having any suicidal thoughts?"

"A few," he admits, knowing I will be worried.

"I will have your dad reach out to Dr. Allen. Then she can call you in a new prescription." *Will this even help? I'm not even there to comfort and help him.*

"I don't want to take medication for the rest of my life!" I can hear desperation, anger, and fear in my son's voice.

"You may have to take medication for a while to help you. It won't be forever." I honestly don't know if he will always have to take antidepressants or not.

"OK," Josh concedes.

"Josh, I love you."

"Love you too, Mom."

I hang up and immediately call Aaron. We still have guardianship of Josh to help with his mental health care. Aaron agrees to get in touch with the psychiatrist and get the prescription. I walk back to the table to eat my dinner, but my appetite left the minute I heard the anguish in Josh's voice. Grant smiles to greet me as I slump into my chair.

"Josh is not doing well." I deliver the news to him.

"I'm here for you, and I will do anything I can to help."

"Thank you. I love you." I see concern in Grant's eyes.

"Are you hungry?" he asks me.

"Not really, but I will try to eat a little." I cut my steak and force myself to chew.

I'm thankful that Josh reached out to me this time. But I feel completely helpless.

After dinner, we step outside, onto the deck. The sun is setting over the Atlantic Ocean. It looks like someone painted gold, orange, and red in long streaks right into the blue, sparkling water. Grant pulls me close to him. The warmth of his body and the strength of his arms give me peace and courage simultaneously.

God, please be with Josh, and surround him with your angels.

I visualize my prayer as a boat setting sail to my son on the other side of the country.

Grant takes my hand and leads me inside.

I feel slightly grounded by his touch, but I want to run, swim, fly off this ship.

I want to be with my son to comfort him. Tears start flowing down my cheeks.

In our room, with Grant's arms around me, I drift off to sleep.

My dreams are not so kind, though.

I'm in dark, murky water. I can't see anything. I feel my panic rise when I feel something near me. I realize it's my son. Opening my mouth to yell out to him, I swallow water. He's drifting away from me.

I start to swim, but I'm not moving forward. I'm not moving at all. It feels as though I'm swimming in mud. There is a ray of light, and I catch a glimpse of my son. I'm not able to reach him.

I'm awakened by a scream. It's my scream. Grant pulls me closer.

"I am here," he whispers to me. "I love you."

If only I could reach my son to help him.

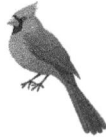

CHAPTER THIRTY-NINE

Hope in Friends

A thousand miles away from you

A broken mess ...

I tried so hard ...

I've lost so much ...

Then I'll see your face ...

You call my name

I come to you in pieces

So you can make me whole

—"Pieces," Red

Josh

I walk to the Golden Gate Bridge and wander through the park. It's twilight, and very few people are around. I keep walking until I get to the foot of the bridge. I walk up the footpath on one side. I didn't really plan to come to the bridge, but I'm having lots of suicidal thoughts.

I should've kept taking my medication.

What is my deal with bridges? This will be the third time I've thought about jumping. That thought alone makes me sad. *Depression has such a hold on me.*

I stand at the top and look out over the water for a long time.

"God, where are you?" I yell out over the sea. It's fifty degrees outside.

Just then I feel a warm breeze. *Could that be God?* I start walking down the footpath on the side of the bridge and back through the park. Luckily, my phone still has some charge. I request an Uber to go back to my apartment. All of a sudden, I feel complete exhaustion.

I feel so alone. I know God saved me again tonight.

I'm thankful for Mom and Dad. They reached out to my therapist in South Carolina. She agreed to Skype me, and she called in a new prescription for me. I'm hopeful it will help me this time. I do like my school, but I'm having trouble concentrating in class.

Two weeks after starting the new medication, I'm starting to feel better. I have good days and bad days. Since moving to San Francisco, I've lost a lot of weight just by walking and eating less. As I climb the hill back to my apartment, my phone starts ringing.

"Hey, Mom," I answer.

"Hi, how are you feeling?" she asks me right away.

"I'm feeling a little better." I can say that truthfully.

"I want to come see you the second weekend in November," Mom states.

"OK, I will be available that weekend. I do have classes on Friday, though."

"I can schedule a flight to get in that morning and do a little sightseeing. Can't wait to see you. Love you."

I really would like to see and talk to her.

"Love you too, Mom." I'm excited she is coming to visit.

I cook eggs for dinner. I do make a very good omelet. Going back to my room, I feel sad again. My roommate, Max, goes home a lot. His family lives in Southern California.

So, I'm alone a lot.

I'm doing homework when Dad calls.

"Hi, Josh, how are you?"

"Hey, Dad, I'm doing better. The medicine is helping this time. Mom called earlier, and she's coming to visit in November."

"That's great. I want to come to see you right before Christmas."

"Sure, you can come in December." They must be worried about me. "Talk to you later."

Did I make the right decision, moving to the other side of the country? *I really do miss Mom and Dad. But I want to continue my classes and make it work here.*

I get ready for bed and pull out my extra blanket. The nights here are getting chillier.

When I open my eyes, it's light out. Wow, I feel so much better after a good night's sleep. My first class isn't until eleven o'clock this morning. I grab a hot tea and a breakfast sandwich from Starbucks on my way to school. *I'm nervous about being early. What will I do?*

A pretty girl, whom I have seen before, smiles as I walk in. Wow, coming in early, and not in a rush, has its advantages.

"Hi, I'm Laura," she says, looking directly at me.

"Josh," I barely get out my name.

Why is it so hard for me to talk to girls? Actually, it's hard for me to talk to anyone.

"When's your first class?" she asks me.

"Not until eleven, but I want to get some work done."

"Oh, good for you." She winks at me. "Hope you get a lot of work done."

"Thank you." I wave to her as I get into the elevator.

I actually get a lot of studying done before my class.

"Hey, Josh, want to go grab lunch together?" Ben, one of my classmates, asks.

"Yeah, sure. That would be great."

Ben and I walk to Chipotle together. I order my favorite salad. We find a spot away from the front door, and he proceeds to tell me about a fun party next weekend.

"Yeah, that sounds really cool." I would like to be able to meet people and hang out.

After lunch, I head back to school for my last class of the day. Laura is back, and I want to ask her so many questions. *Where are you from? What do you like to do for fun? Tell me about your family.*

I bravely walk toward the front desk, where she's sitting.

"Hey, Josh, what kind of music do you like?" Laura asks me first.

"All kinds. Well, maybe not country."

"Oh, cool. Me too," she responds. "Maybe we can catch my favorite band, Seven Days Straight?"

"Yes, I would really like that." *Wow, did she just ask me out?*

"Awesome—they play a lot around here. Have a good class."

"OK, catch you later." I turn to go to the elevator.

Just then, I think of Carrie.

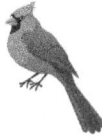

CHAPTER FORTY

Preparing for Connection

Maria

I'm so excited to see Josh. My heart aches as I realize how much I miss him. I've been to San Francisco before. Audra and I went two years ago to look at colleges for her.

It's going to be colder there than it is here in Charleston. I pack several of my favorite sweaters and a black wrap.

I feel fear rise in me, knowing that Josh will be as depressed as he has been in the past. I push the fear away and think about hugging my wonderful son.

Sitting down with Grant, we research some fun things to do in San Francisco. I really want to take Josh on a sunset sailing cruise. I find the perfect trip and send him a text to see which day would be best for him.

Hi, Josh. Looking forward to seeing you this weekend.

Me too, he texts right back.

Would Saturday night or Sunday night be better for a sunset sailing trip?

Several minutes pass, and no response. I distract myself by looking at other excursions.

Sunday night would work, Josh writes back.

OK, I will look at what's available.

Mom, I have a lot of schoolwork. I have an early day tomorrow.

Sleep well. I love you.

Love you too, Mom.

I book the sunset cruise for this Sunday. I continue to look at other excursions. I would really like to go to Alcatraz. Best to wait to book that until I confirm with Josh tomorrow. I realize I have been on the computer for almost two hours.

"I'm going to turn in, sweetheart," I say, kissing Grant on the lips. He is staying with me for a few days; we have been looking for townhomes not far from where I live to rent together.

"OK, beautiful, I will be up soon."

I pull out my favorite silk pajamas. After washing my face, I start rolling my clothes to pack in my suitcase. Ten minutes later, I'm almost done packing. I like having time to add the last-minute things.

I'm so grateful and happy that I get to see Josh soon.

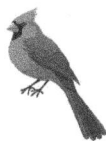

CHAPTER FORTY-ONE

Moments of Possibility

There's another world inside of me ...
There's secrets in this life ...
And somewhere in this darkness
There's a light ...
Or maybe I'm just blind ...
Hold me when I'm scared
And love me when I'm gone.
—"When I'm Gone," 3 Doors Down

Josh

I'm happy Mom is coming to visit, and I'm upset at the same time. Not with her; with me. *Why can't I get my life on track?* I'm not eating well, and I can't sleep consistently. The medicine is starting to help this time, and I have really good days. But then, the next day, the terrible thoughts return.

I made the decision to come out to California to get away. I really needed a fresh start. *I want to be able to do it on my own. Can I do it on my own? I realize now that it's OK for me to accept help from my family.*

I will have a good time with Mom. I want to eat at some of the great restaurants and explore San Francisco.

I dress quickly, putting on the same pants I've worn for three days. I'll have to do laundry after class. As I head down the hill toward school, I know San Francisco is a great city for me.

"Hi, Josh," Laura greets me as I enter the school.

"Hey, Laura. How are you?"

"I'm great, thank you for asking." She smiles at me. I love her smile.

As I head upstairs to class, I think of Carrie again. *I have not heard from her in a while. To be fair, I have not called or texted her either. I wonder how she's been.* My thoughts are interrupted by the teacher starting class.

Classes fly by today, and I feel good with how well I'm doing in all of them. Ben and I study together after class again. Studying with someone helps keep me focused.

"Hey, man, whatcha doing this weekend?" Ben asks me as we gather our things.

"My mom is actually coming into town," I tell him.

"Oh, that's cool. Moms are the best."

I nod, knowing he's right. I have a flood of memories of Mom. *She really loves me.*

"See you tomorrow, Josh." Ben heads out the door.

"Yes, see you then." I take a few more minutes to gather my books.

I begin the climb up the several blocks to my apartment building. I make chicken noodle soup from a can for dinner. As I get back to my room with my soup bowl, the phone rings.

"Hi, Carrie, it's so good to hear from you." *I wonder why she is calling me.*

"How have you been, Josh?" she asks me right away.

"Pretty good. I really like it here in San Francisco. You're welcome to visit anytime."

"Oh, maybe—we always have fun together," Carrie responds.

"How have you been?" I realize we have not talked since we broke up.

"I'm doing great. I have thought about you a lot lately."

Hearing Carrie's voice really chokes me up. "Me too. I wanted to text you the other day."

I try to keep the conversation going. "My mom is coming to visit this weekend. I'm excited to see her. I will let you know how her visit goes." *Why did I say I would tell her how it goes? We don't talk every day.*

"Please say hi to your mom for me," Carrie continues. "I have missed you, Josh."

"I've missed you too. It's good to hear from you. Good night."

I stare at the phone as the call ends. I open my pictures on my phone and look at our photos. I really do miss Carrie. Maybe, after Mom and Dad visit, I will ask if she wants to visit over the Christmas break. The thought of her coming to see me makes me really happy.

I hope that she says yes to visiting.

Today was a good day.

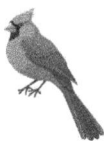

CHAPTER FORTY-TWO

Visiting Josh

Maria

Why do I choose early flights? I know it's to make the most of my vacation, but getting to the airport at 5:00 a.m. is a bit crazy.

Grant walks me in and checks my bag. He wanted to come with me, but he is finishing up a big work project.

"I love you so much." I kiss him on the cheek.

"I love you too. Please text me when you land."

"I will see you in five days." I hug him goodbye.

Grant kisses me, and I feel it everywhere. I compose myself with a smile and blow him a kiss goodbye. I get through security quickly and go in search of coffee. The warm, dark, rich coffee gives me the wake-up I really need. I browse through the new books at the bookstore, looking for something for the long flight. I love reading, but I know my mind will wander. I end up choosing the latest *Cosmopolitan* magazine and a pack of gum.

We board early. I am thankful and ready to start my trip.

I awaken to a kind older flight attendant asking if I would like something to drink.

"Coffee, please, with two cream and no sugar."

I look at my phone and realize I've been asleep for an hour. When the flight attendant returns with my hot coffee, I sip it cautiously and peruse my *Cosmopolitan*. I really need to be distracted from worrying about Josh.

"We are beginning our descent into the Bay Area. Please put your seats in the upright position, and stow all your belongings," the pilot announces, waking me again.

Wow, I slept almost the entire flight.

Hi, I just landed. Love you, I text Grant.

He texts me back. *Glad you made it safe. Love you more.*

After getting my bag, I go in search of the metro to take to my hotel. The hotel I chose is located in Chinatown, close to Josh's apartment. I thought it would be fun to try a hotel in Chinatown. The atmosphere there is exciting, with beautiful Chinese lanterns hanging above and twirling in the wind.

I find the hotel and check in. The room is horrible—it's the size of a hostel room. And it's dark and has an awful musty smell. I walk out of the room and go down the elevator and into the lobby. I ask the woman at the counter for a full refund. I pull out my phone and use my favorite hotel app to find a better place to stay. I find the hotel that Audra and I stayed in two years ago. They have availability, and it's $100 cheaper. *I should've just booked it in the first place.*

After I get settled at the Breakers Hotel, I head downstairs to get lunch at the hotel restaurant. I order an iced tea and a salad and just relax. Josh is still in class, so I will go to see him around six o'clock this evening. Then we can go together to a local restaurant for dinner.

First, I take an Uber to go and see Lombard Street. It's so crazy that they built a road that zigzags like that. Afterward, I wander around the Hyde Street Pier. I then stumble upon the Buena Vista Cafe and decide to go in. The café is famous for its Irish coffee. I splurge and order one, and I'm immediately warmed up.

Leaving the café, I walk some more, but my boots are starting to hurt my feet. I open the Uber app and get a ride back to the hotel to change for dinner. The hotel is offering happy hour in the parlor, and I ask for a pinot noir. Sitting down, I feel exhausted. But I'm also excited to see my son. I have a flashback to the trip to Atlanta. I tear up, remembering Josh walking away from me. *I want this trip to be relaxing and fun.*

After finishing my wine, I walk into the lobby and order an Uber. Arriving ten minutes later at Josh's apartment, I get out of the car and walk up the steps. I ring the intercom, and Josh says he will be right down.

Josh greets me with a huge smile. He's lost a lot of weight, but he looks healthy.

"Hi, Mom." He gives me a big hug.

"I'm so happy to see you." I tear up.

"Me too," Josh responds. "Wanna see my room?"

"Yes, I would love to." I follow him up a flight of stairs. His room is a good size, and it has a fireplace.

"We don't use it," he speaks up, as if he read my mind. "My roommate is not here much, and I don't want to start a fire just for me."

"I will have to send you some pictures," I remark, noting how bare the walls look.

"Sure, I have not had much time."

"Ready to go get dinner?" I ask.

"Yes, I'm starving." Josh grabs his jacket, and we walk out of his apartment building.

It's a lot further to the restaurant I chose than I expected. Josh proudly leads the way, so I continue on for a while. But then, I spot a seafood restaurant on the way. We stop to look at the menu.

"Yeah, this place looks good, Mom," Josh comments.

The wait is not long, and the food is delicious. However, the conversation with my son is the best part of the night.

Josh shares with me that he wants to be able to start doing things on his own. He really loves California. He's finally meeting friends and doing better in school. I love listening to everything he tells me.

After dinner, I put in for a multi-stop Uber so we can both head to bed.

"Thanks, Mom. You must be pretty tired too."

"I am—we can both get to bed early. Tomorrow will be fun."

"Alcatraz should be cool," Josh adds.

The Uber drops Josh off first. "Bye, sweetheart."

"Bye, Mom. See you in the morning."

I watch Josh walk in the door to his apartment building. The Uber takes me back to my hotel, and I head right to my room.

God, thank you for a safe trip and for time with my son today.

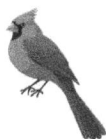

CHAPTER FORTY-THREE

My Mom

For you, there'll be no more crying ...
Because I feel that when I'm with you
It's alright ...
To you, I'll give the world ...
And the songbirds are singing ...
And I love you, I love you, I love you
—"Songbird," Fleetwood Mac

Josh

It was really great to see Mom last night, but I honestly don't want to get out of bed this morning. *She wants to go to Alcatraz. Really, Mom? That sounds very depressing.* I know she thinks seeing the sights around San Francisco will be good for me, but I really just want to sleep.

I read Mom's text. *Good morning, hope you slept well. I will be there in an hour. Would you like a green tea and a breakfast sandwich from Starbucks?*

Morning. Yeah, thanks.

So, I drag myself out of bed and head to the bathroom. I splash water on my face and brush my teeth. Back in my room, I put on the same clothes I wore yesterday. I will accept Mom's offer to get me new clothes today. I told her that since losing weight, most of my clothes don't fit anymore.

"Morning," I say to her as I get in the Uber.

"Morning, Josh. Here's your green tea and breakfast."

"Thanks, Mom." She knows that I don't like coffee.

Waiting in line to take the ferry to Alcatraz, I look around at the other people. *Why are all these people in line to go and see this depressing place?* Dealing with depression and anxiety, I avoid places with too many people. Over-the-top energy and excessive talking are too much for me.

The ferry ride over is uneventful. Mom and I get right off and start walking around on our own. It's an eerie place, and the morning fog adds to the eeriness. I will admit that I'm a little intrigued at how the prisoners lived on this creepy island. Right then, I feel a chill.

The island's a lot bigger than I thought. Mom reads the placards at each stop. The one fact that's interesting is that the prison guards had apartments, and their whole families lived on the island. Kids even had school here. Now that would be scary.

Next, we go inside the prison to look around. *It's dark and cold. I feel like the walls are closing in on me. I'm done with this depressing place.*

Mom senses it and suggests, "Why don't we head back and take the next ferry?"

"OK," I murmur, and we walk back down to the dock and board the ferry.

"Would you like some hot chocolate to warm up?" Mom asks me.

"Sure, that would be good." She hands me a hot chocolate and sits down next to me.

We enjoy our hot drinks and the quiet ferry ride back.

Back at the port, we get another Uber and head to the mall. Mom suggests we try American Eagle. We check the directory to find that store. Trying on new pants, I realize I need more than one pair. Mom buys me a warm coat, two pairs of pants, three shirts, and a new hat too.

"I really appreciate all of this, Mom."

"You're so welcome, Josh."

"For lunch, can I show you this new place that has great poke bowls?" I suggest.

"Sounds wonderful. Let's go and get two bowls." Mom follows me.

I order the steak bowl, and Mom orders the tuna bowl.

"So, where to next?" Mom asks.

"Mom, would it be OK if you took me back to my place to rest for a while?"

"Of course," Mom acquiesces as she looks away.

I know she's disappointed. But I really need to lie down.

I wake up three hours later and remember Mom is in town.

Hi. How was your afternoon? I text her.

I went to the Japanese Tea Garden, and it was beautiful.

Can we meet for dinner? I'm really hungry.

Of course. I just got back to my hotel.

Just let me know when is good for you, Mom, I text, hoping it's soon.

I can meet you in an hour.

After I take a hot shower, I put on my new jeans and one of my new shirts.

I'm so grateful for the new clothes.

Mom is outside one hour later, and we ride together to a nearby restaurant.

"Mom, thank you for this morning, my new clothes, and understanding."

"Of course. I love you. And I'm so happy to be here with you."

We enjoy a delicious dinner of sushi, pad thai, and red curry. *Mom can be annoying at times, asking me constantly how I am. Then at other times, like tonight, she just gets me.*

"Night, Josh. I had a great day with you today."

"Me too." I hug her. Mom understood me today. She knew when I needed space.

God, thank you for my mom.

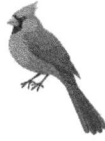

CHAPTER FORTY-FOUR

Quiet Spaces

Maria

I wake up super early. Oh, right: It's ten o'clock in the morning in Charleston. I'm not able to fall back asleep. I decide to go and explore more of San Francisco. I start walking toward the Ferry Building. Twelve blocks later, I finally arrive. It's so foggy this morning; I can barely see the harbor. Inside the building, there are many local restaurants, all under one roof. I send a text to Josh to ask if he would like me to bring him breakfast again.

Hi Josh, good morning.

Hi, Mom, he texts right back.

Would you like a hot tea and a bagel?

Yes, thanks.

OK, I will be over in half an hour. I sit down to enjoy my breakfast.

The sun is trying to break through the fog. I enjoy my croissant and coffee and a quiet moment for myself. I want to be there for Josh today.

Dear God, please help Josh to feel better, and please be with both of us today.

I go in search of green tea and a bagel for Josh. Then I grab an Uber and head to his apartment. Josh is waiting outside, and he greets me with a big smile as he gets in the car.

"Morning, Josh." I'm so thankful he's in good spirits.

"Hi, Mom, thank you." Josh accepts the tea and bagel.

I ask the Uber driver to take us to Twin Peaks. We wind up the hill to the view at the top. Getting out, we both begin to walk to the edge to look over. All of San Francisco spreads out below us. The Golden Gate Bridge looks like a toy bridge, but it's still distinguishable. We climb up higher on one peak and can see 360 degrees.

It really is breathtaking. I feel such peace and take in the beauty that spreads below us. And, in this moment, I feel connected to my son.

Josh tolerates a few selfies of us. I take way too many pictures of the scenic view. Josh agrees to walk through Golden Gate Park, so the next Uber driver takes us there.

"So, how have you been doing in school?" I ask as we walk through the park.

"I've been doing well in school, and I like all of my classes."

"Oh, that's good." I wait for him to continue.

"It's just hard when I don't feel like getting out of bed."

"Are you still having trouble sleeping?" I ask, concerned again.

"Yeah, I'm up most of the night."

"So the sleep medicine doesn't help?" I wonder if we will ever find the right sleep medicine for him. I want to help Josh with his sleep and depression.

"Dr. Allen just gave me a new one, and I sleep a little better sometimes."

We walk in silence for a while. I know that the silence between us is a bridge to understanding each other better.

"Hey, Mom, can I go back to lie down now?" Josh asks, breaking the silence.

"Sure thing." I open the app to request another Uber driver.

This driver talks nonstop. He tells us he's a dad making extra money on the weekend. I share with him that I'm visiting from Charleston.

"Oh, I have always wanted to visit the South," he exclaims.

"I've been there sixteen years, but I'm originally from Pennsylvania." I continue the conversation.

"I have family in Philly—I want to visit there too. Hey, would you both like to go down Lombard Street?"

I'm about to say yes, but I see that Josh is getting very irritated.

"Oh, I have seen it. Thank you," I respond.

"It's right here. Just two more blocks."

I want to say no, thank you, but I don't want to be rude. Josh has closed his eyes. I want Josh to be happy, but I really want to drive down the famous serpentine street. Before I speak up, we are at the top of the road, committed to heading down since it's one way. My son is quiet and visibly upset. I realize that I cannot influence his mood, and I just enjoy the twists and turns.

When we arrive at Josh's apartment, he gets out after saying a quick goodbye.

"Would you still like to meet for dinner in a few hours?" I ask him hopefully.

"Sure, Mom," he responds and closes the car door.

The Uber driver talks all the way back to my hotel. I thank him for everything and get out of the car. I head upstairs to my room and decide to take a nap too. I put on a big fluffy robe and climb under the covers.

I wake up almost two hours later. I guess I'm still adjusting to the time difference. After a hot shower, I pull out my black jeans, green sweater, and black boots. I venture downstairs to ask the concierge for restaurant recommendations. After I pick one that I like, he calls to make a reservation for me.

The hotel is having a happy hour in the library again. I have some time before going to meet Josh. So I walk into the library and get a glass of pinot noir. I find a comfy green velvet armchair and listen to the musician playing Broadway tunes on the piano. The roaring fire in the fireplace, the red wine, and the piano tempt me back to sleep.

A nice couple from Chicago sit down on the couch near me. Striking up a conversation with them keeps me awake.

I share that I'm here visiting my son. They tell me all about their grown children and grandchildren, whom they are here visiting. Time slips by quickly, and I have to abruptly excuse myself. Fortunately, the Uber driver is close by.

We arrive at Josh's place a few minutes later. He's outside waiting and jumps right into the car. I have already asked the driver to take us to the restaurant. Josh is in much better spirits. Tonight, we are going to one of the best restaurants in Chinatown.

Josh speaks up when we get out of the car. "Mom, thank you."

"For what?" I ask, wondering.

"Just for understanding that I need time alone sometimes."

"Of course—I have many days when I want to be alone," I confess.

"You do?" he asks incredulously.

"Yes, definitely! Taking time to be alone and taking care of yourself are both very important to your emotional and mental health." I can see Josh contemplating what I just shared.

We order drinks and appetizers before our dinner. I look at Josh. *God has blessed me with such a wonderful son.*

CHAPTER FORTY-FOUR

We both share our main courses and talk about our day tomorrow.

"Would you like to see my school?" Josh asks.

"Of course. We can go in the morning." I'm excited he wants to show me his school.

The waiter brings the check, and I pull out my phone to get another Uber.

Maybe I should have rented a car.

We ride in silence.

When we pull up to Josh's apartment, I get out briefly to say good night.

"Good night, Josh." I give him a big hug. "See you in the morning."

"Night, Mom." He heads inside his building.

I get back in the car to head back to my hotel.

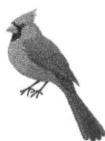

CHAPTER FORTY-FIVE

Big Red Giant

Josh

I wake up, and the sun is shining through the window. I slept all night and I'm looking forward to spending this last day with Mom. We're going to walk around so I can show her my school.

"Morning," I say, greeting Mom outside my apartment building.

"How did you sleep last night?" she questions me.

"I slept much better. How about you, Mom?"

"I slept great, thanks for asking me." She looks touched I asked.

We walk downhill, toward my school. It's six blocks straight downhill. In Charleston, everything is flat. It took me several weeks to get used to all the hills in San Francisco.

Washington Square is already decorated for Christmas—it's only the second weekend in November. Mom asks if she can take a picture of me in front of the tree. I agree, feeling uplifted by the festive atmosphere. We continue walking two more blocks, and I take Mom into the main school building to show her some of my classrooms. I love showing Mom around—especially the lab where I spend a lot of my time.

My stomach rumbles as we are leaving the building.

"Let's head to Fisherman's Wharf and get a late lunch," Mom suggests.

"Yes, I'm really hungry," I confess.

The weather is nice, so we walk. On the way, I see the Verizon store.

"Hey, Mom, could we run in and get a case for my new phone?"

"Sure thing." She follows me into the store.

Half an hour later, I have a new case, a screen protector, and an extra charger.

I'm definitely ready to eat now. Fisherman's Wharf is packed. We find a fish place that has a self-service counter. Mom gets fish chowder, and I get fish-and-chips. I'm starting to feel irritable; maybe I have low blood sugar. I am shoveling my food into my mouth so fast, I have to keep reminding myself to slow down. Most likely, I'm just getting frustrated with all the people around. I have never liked crowds, but I especially hate being around a lot of people when I'm down.

Mom senses that I'm uncomfortable. We eat in silence. I'm so thankful that Mom is starting to understand me now.

"How about we walk toward that park over there, away from everyone?" she offers.

I nod and get up to throw out my lunch trash. We head to the park. Sitting and watching the dogs play helps relax me a little.

"Our cruise on the harbor is in an hour," Mom reminds me.

I don't respond, still feeling very agitated. I close my eyes and let the sun warm my face. Maybe it can give me energy and help me feel better.

"I'm going to go and get a keychain for AJ." Mom stands to walk toward the wharf.

"OK, I will be here." Mom leaves, and I'm happy to be alone.

I must have drifted off to sleep. Mom is back, sitting next to me and smiling.

"You have a good nap?" she asks me.

"I do feel better."

"Josh, I know you hate crowds. The cruise will only have about forty people on board."

"OK, Mom." I say what she wants to hear. I'm just ready to go home.

How can my day start off so well and then get like this?

Mom gets up, and I follow her back to the pier. When we get in line for the cruise, it looks like more than forty people. I look out over the water to keep myself calm. The weather starts getting much cooler. As we start boarding the boat, I head straight inside to get away from people, and Mom follows me.

The captain gives us some instructions as the boat leaves the dock. It gets really foggy and cold, even inside. The captain indicates that the blue jackets around the boat are for us to use; Mom hands me one to put on. People keep coming aboard, and it's getting even more crowded, with people in puffy blue jackets all around me.

"You want to go and stand on the upper deck?" Mom looks at me.

"No, I'm going to stay here."

"OK, I will be back," she says, heading up the stairs.

She is back five minutes later.

"It's freezing, and the fog is too thick to see anything," she explains to me.

We're heading toward the Golden Gate Bridge. The captain says it will take about twenty minutes.

I know I'm being difficult, but I want this ridiculous cruise to be over. Mom and I sit in silence as the boat chugs along through the San Francisco Bay. Just as the engine turns off, the sky clears. We can see the bridge through the windows.

"I'm going to go back up to see." Mom stands.

"OK, I will be up in a bit."

As Mom goes up again, I pout some more. After five minutes, I decide to go up and look around. It's absolutely beautiful; the sun is setting behind the bridge. We're so close, it looks like a big red giant. Everyone is taking pictures, including Mom. I relax a little and enjoy the view.

"Could we get a picture together?" Mom asks me hesitantly.

I know how much she likes to capture memories in pictures. "Sure."

We're able to enjoy the view for another half hour. Then the engine roars back to life, and we head back toward the city.

I continue to enjoy the view on the upper deck; I'm thankful Mom and I can be together without needing to talk. The past few days have been challenging for me. Mom showed me much of the city that I now call home. She also showed me that she understands and loves me.

My heart feels full. I feel that love for myself grow. *Maybe healing starts with self-love.*

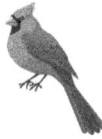

CHAPTER FORTY-SIX

Bridges of Love

Maria

I'm enjoying my last day with Josh. I know that he has been agitated and even uncomfortable many times over the past few days. But I honestly think that he enjoyed getting out to see San Francisco with me. The cruise started off a little rough; the weather shifted, and it was so foggy and cold as we set out into the harbor. Josh and I put on the down jackets they provided for us.

I make my way onto the upper deck, but it's freezing, and with the fog, I can't see anything. I quickly retreat below and go in search of coffee, but they only have decaf left. I opt for a glass of red wine.

Josh seems so unhappy, and he's super quiet. I'm frustrated that he doesn't seem to be appreciating the cruise. *I want to be sensitive to his struggles, but sometimes I want him to just enjoy.*

Another fifteen minutes pass, and rays of light come in through the windows.

I carefully navigate around the people and emerge back up on the upper deck. The view is breathtaking: Orange, gold, mauve, and pink streaks emblazon the sky. The Golden Gate Bridge towers above the boat; I'm mesmerized by its beauty.

Josh surprises me a few minutes later by joining me. We stand in silence and deep appreciation. He seems to soften and take it all in. I take several pictures and ask him to pose for a picture with me.

"Thanks for taking a picture with me. I'm going below for a bit."

"OK, Mom. I'm going to stay here."

I look back to see him walking around to take in the view. *Maybe Josh just needs to navigate his emotions in his own way.*

"God, thank you," I whisper out to sea.

The sun is going down as I venture below to warm up. A few brave souls stay where they are, including Josh. Eventually, I go back up and stand next to my son as we head back in.

Another ten minutes later, we're back at the dock.

We all disembark, leaving the jackets and extending our thanks to the captain and the crew. Taking our last Uber of the day, we head back to Josh's apartment.

"Mom, I want to thank you for this weekend."

"You're welcome—I enjoyed our visit. I love you."

"Love you too, Mom. Bye." He gives me a big hug and stands at the door to his apartment to wave goodbye.

I wave too, as a tear slips down my cheek.

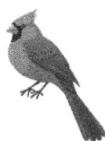

CHAPTER FORTY-SEVEN

Tentative Steps

Climbing up on Solsbury Hill ...
Wind was blowing, time stood still ...
Came in close, I heard a voice ...
I had to listen, had no choice ...
My heart going "Boom, boom, boom" ...
"Grab your things, I've come to take you home"
—"Solsbury Hill," Peter Gabriel

Josh

Now what do I do? Mom has gone home to Charleston. I realize now that I'm a little homesick.

I have classes and see people, but I'm still mostly alone. I keep to myself because I don't think anyone will really like me; I can be very moody. Mom says I am kind, perceptive, and a good friend. She encourages me to meet new people. *OK, Mom. I will make an effort to talk to more people at school.*

I really want to go back to sleep, but I force myself to get up. I head out to get tea and a breakfast sandwich on the way.

The really nice girl at Starbucks greets me by name. "Hi, Josh."

"Hi—green tea and an egg sandwich, please?" I give her my order.

"Sure thing."

I hand her my card, and I wait. After I get my breakfast sandwich and my tea, I head out the door toward my school. I get to my class just in time. Luckily, I only have two classes back-to-back, and they're both easy.

After I leave school for the day, I decide to explore San Francisco. I download a map of the city and head to a park nearby. I realize I have stayed in a one-mile radius pretty much since I got here. With Mom, I explored more of the city, and now I want to see more.

When I first came here, I did visit the Golden Gate Park. It was then that I decided I wanted to live here.

Getting up from the park bench, I start heading toward the Ferry Building. I usually don't notice other people around me. This time, I look up while I'm walking; it's amazing to see so many different types of people.

I must have walked twenty blocks when I finally arrive at my destination. Once inside, I go in search of lemonade. I don't normally drink it, but I'm really thirsty and want lemonade. I order a large one and head outside to find a bench overlooking the water. After going to Alcatraz by ferry and on the sunset cruise with Mom, the harbor now intrigues me. It's a really big harbor, yet the water is calm and welcoming today.

I finish my lemonade while walking through another park. This park allows me to see spectacular views of the water. After another hour passes, I start heading back toward my street. I spent the afternoon alone, but I feel like I learned more about a friend—San Francisco is my new friend.

Right before I get to my apartment, I head into the local market and buy a sandwich and a bottle of water. I will have an early dinner tonight. When I get to my room, my roommate is back. He's home after being away for the weekend.

"How was your weekend, Max?" I ask him.

"It was good; how about yours?" Max responds.

"Good—my mom and I had a really great time touring San Francisco."

"It really is a great city." He shares his thoughts.

"Yeah, I think so too." I recall all I have seen and done the past five days.

Max and I end up hanging out together. He offers me a beer and some of the pizza he ordered. I will save my sandwich for lunch tomorrow. We end up watching *The Avengers*.

Hanging out with Max, I realize we have a lot of things in common. He was a goalie for his high school soccer team, and he has two brothers and a sister too. It's great to learn more about Max, and I feel accepted by him. Meeting new people will stretch me past my comfort zone, yet it will offer me many more opportunities.

I'm tired of being sad and depressed, and I'm definitely tired of sitting home alone.

Today is the beginning of a new me—having fun and enjoying my life.

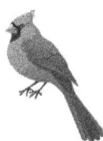

CHAPTER FORTY-EIGHT

Finding Joy

Maria

Going back to work today is especially hard. My thoughts are still with Josh. There were many times when I could see his anxiety and feel his sadness. But he seemed better when I left. I find comfort in knowing that Aaron is going out to visit him just before Christmas. I really hate the idea of Josh being alone for Christmas.

How can I make Josh feel the magic of Christmas? I decide to send him gift cards for each of the twelve days of Christmas. Focusing on finding the best gift cards for him will direct my focus from worry to joy.

At lunch, I walk to the grocery store. I buy six gift cards: two for the movie theater—Josh likes movies but would not buy movie tickets for himself; two Visa gift cards, to buy more clothes or whatever he wants; an Uber card—that way he can get around San Francisco; and a gift card for Target. I will buy the rest of the gift cards later this week. I also pick up funny Christmas cards and stamps. I grab a Cobb salad and check out.

Aaron calls as I walk back to work. "How was your visit to see Josh?"

"Hi, we had a really great visit together. We went to Alcatraz, Golden Gate Park, and Twin Peaks, and took a sunset cruise from Pier 39 to the Golden Gate Bridge. Josh enjoyed most of it, but he did seem agitated on the boat and walking through Golden Gate Park. I bought him a new coat, jeans, shirts, and food to stock up his fridge and pantry. We ran out of time, but I'm sure that Josh would like to ride a cable car when you go to visit."

"OK, I will start to plan my visit. Thanks for letting me know how he's feeling and what you did together."

I end the call with Aaron and quickly eat my salad in the break room.

The afternoon goes by pretty fast; I'm concentrating better and get a lot of work done. Heading home, I listen to my favorite country station. After dinner, I write the first Christmas card to let Josh know he will be getting twelve gift cards for Christmas. I smile as I tuck the gift cards and greeting cards into my leather tote bag. I head upstairs to take a hot bubble bath. The hot water relaxes my muscles. *I really need to take better care of myself.*

I say good night to AJ and Grant.

"Good night—I love you. I'm going to bed early," I tell Grant.

"Good night, beautiful." I kiss him and head to bed.

Waking up, I see the sun coming in through the blinds. I slept straight through the night; I really needed that sleep. *I feel like a new woman.*

My favorite French coffee smells and tastes delicious this morning. I grab my ham and Swiss cheese sandwich and add an apple to my lunch bag. I feel much better equipped to face the day than I did yesterday.

When I get to work, I find a text from Josh on my phone.

Hi, Mom.

Hi, Josh. How are you?

I feel better. I want to thank you again for a great weekend.

You're so welcome. It was great to see you.

I'm so thankful to you and Dad for being there for me.

You know we always will be.

I know, thank you. I love you.

I love you too.

I exhale. *God, please continue to surround my son with your angels.*

My day goes by quickly since I'm extremely busy. On my way home from work, I stop at the grocery store and buy steaks, potatoes, salad, and a bottle of cabernet sauvignon. I'm going to make a nice dinner for Grant. AJ is having dinner with his girlfriend and her parents. I'm looking forward to an evening that Grant and I can spend together.

The house is quiet when I get home. I change into my rose cashmere sweater and black cashmere joggers. I have time to marinate the steak and prepare the potatoes.

As I am setting the table, Grant walks in. He greets me with a passionate kiss.

"Well, hello," I say, blushing.

"What's all this?" he asks with amusement.

"Dinner for you and me." I feel my body relax.

"Ah, that sounds perfect. Let me change, and I will start the grill."

We cook together and set out the food. I light the candles on the table as Grant opens the bottle of wine. We laugh and talk over dinner about the food, decorations, and music for our wedding celebration.

Leaving the dishes, Grant takes me by my hand and leads me upstairs. I really have missed his touch. We lie in each other's arms for a while. He asks about Josh and my trip. I share with him all that we did and the joys and my fears. Grant just listens and holds me tighter.

I feel so loved by Grant. *His love is the strength I need. I'm blessed that he's in my life.*

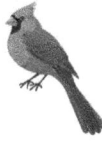

CHAPTER FORTY-NINE

Social Courage

Josh

I'm up early this morning and quickly dress for school. Locking my door, I shiver in the cold San Francisco air. I button my coat to my neck and go in search of hot tea. I've been trying all different kinds of green tea. I decide to order a matcha tea. It's good but not my favorite.

Today is the last day of classes before finals. My first semester went by fast. As I walk in the front door of the school, Laura is there at the desk.

"Good morning," she greets me with a big smile.

"Hi, morning." I walk up to the desk.

"Would you like to come to a Christmas party this Friday?" Laura asks me.

"Sure," I say, as coolly as I can.

"My roommates and I have an annual ugly Christmas sweater party," she continues.

"I'm sure I can find an ugly sweater I can wear." I chuckle.

"Glad you can come." Laura winks at me.

"Thanks for inviting me. See you later." I walk toward the elevator to go to my last class. *Being invited out by Laura has really cheered me up.*

I barely hear the professor's lecture, as I'm thinking about the party and Laura. I'm so excited to find an ugly Christmas sweater that I rush out of school. I pull out my phone to google the closest Goodwill, and I walk the ten blocks to the store. The store is in several sections: donated clothing and art, kitchen items, and some furniture. I walk to the men's area. It takes several minutes, but I find the perfect ugly sweater; it's dark blue with creepy snowmen all over it. I purchase it for three bucks and go in search of lunch.

Max and I are going to the library after lunch to study for exams. I grab a poke bowl and water at one of my favorite restaurants. The library is not too far from the restaurant.

Max is waiting for me in the lobby.

"Hey, Max."

"Hey—I found a table next to a window." He leads the way.

We study all afternoon. It's helpful to ask each other questions. I will do well on this exam on Friday. We study for two hours and then walk back to our apartment together.

"I'll get the mail," I tell Max.

"OK, I'm heading up to the room."

I have a Christmas card from Mom. She sent me an Uber gift card.

"For the twelve days of Christmas," she wrote on the card. Cool. I like the idea of getting eleven more gift cards.

Max is going to a movie tonight with another friend. He invited me, but I really want some time alone. I like spending time with other people, but I realize I have to find a balance. *If I choose to spend time alone, the choice makes it better.*

I read for a while for my other class, but I can't keep my eyes open. I decide to head to bed early and get a good night's sleep.

Mom has bought me more melatonin. I take two pills and fall right to sleep.

I don't wake up until seven o'clock the next morning. Wow, I feel great after an uninterrupted night's sleep. I get dressed, grab a protein bar and my coat, and head out the front door.

It's easier walking downhill six blocks, and I get to the school right at eight o'clock.

I need to work on my end-of-year project, and I have two final exams. There's a different student at the front desk whom I don't know.

I wave at them and head up to the second floor. It's so quiet, and I get a lot of work done.

"Hi, how are you?" I turn around to see Laura coming into the lab.

"Hi, morning. I'm doing great. How are you?" I ask her.

"I'm a little tired today. I stayed up too late last night."

"Do you have the same project for programming?" I ask curiously.

"Yes, I have a lot to work on. I will be here in the lab most of the day."

"Me too," I offer in support.

Laura gets her computer turned on and pulls out her notebooks.

"I'm going to get a drink downstairs. Can I get you anything?" I ask her.

"Sure, I would love a Diet Coke. Thank you."

I head to the lounge on the first floor. I'm so glad I have change left over from lunch yesterday. Putting the correct change in, I get an iced tea for me and a Diet Coke for Laura. I take the stairs back to the lab.

"Thank you," Laura says as I set the can on her desk.

"You're welcome." I smile in reply.

We both work in silence for the next hour. Laura looks up from her computer and laughs.

"What's so funny?" I laugh when I hear her laugh.

"I was remembering last year's Christmas party. So glad you can come this year."

"It sounds fun. I'm looking forward to it." *I am so happy she invited me.*

"Later today, I'm making a music playlist. Any song requests?" she asks.

"I like most music," I share with her.

"I'd better try to get some more programming done. Sorry to keep distracting you."

I want to tell her she can distract me anytime, but I keep it to myself.

Several other people come in, and the lab gets really noisy. I've worked for hours, and I'm ready to go. I walk over to Laura, and she looks up.

"You heading out?" she asks, bemused.

"Yeah, I have been here for five hours. I did get a lot done," I tell her.

"That's great. I hope to get more done this afternoon."

"Hope you do. See you Friday." *I'm really looking forward to seeing her at the party.*

I go in search of a Chick-fil-A and get a spicy chicken sandwich. Later this afternoon, I'm meeting Max again at the library. It's really cold outside, and I'm so thankful that Mom bought me a warmer coat and hat.

I walk the several blocks from the restaurant back to the library. The fresh air helps give me a second wind.

Max is at our usual table. I spend the rest of the afternoon studying and thinking about Laura. The next two days are going to be long. I want my exams and final lab project to be done already.

"Wanna go hear my friend play at a local bar tonight?" Max asks.

"Yeah, that sounds great. Where is it?" I question him.

"It's not too far from school—in the theater district."

"After the library, we can grab pizza for dinner," I add.

"Sounds good. We can change clothes and head that way," Max continues.

Music at a local bar is not really my scene, but I'm done studying and working on my project for the day. *I also need something to keep my mind off Laura.*

I get my favorite—Hawaiian pizza and a beer. Max gets a pepperoni pizza and a light beer. After devouring our pizza, we quickly change at the apartment. We walk downhill to the pub; I suggest taking an Uber back home later.

The bar smells of whiskey and smoke—a combination of cigarettes, cigars, and weed.

Max's friend and his band are pretty good. They sing a combination of pop and rock.

"They're really good," Max keeps saying all night.

I nod. We both take turns going to the bar.

I have a good time, and I only think of Laura once.

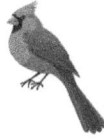

CHAPTER FIFTY

Scattered Celebrations

Maria

Thank goodness it's Friday; I'm really thankful that today is my last day of work for two weeks. I took off Christmas vacation through the New Year. And Audra is coming home today.

At work, my mind wanders all day—thinking about Josh. I will call him at lunch to see how he's doing. *I really don't like that he will be by himself for Christmas this year.*

The morning drags on and on and on. Finally, the chicken salad croissant I ordered for lunch is delivered. I head into the break room to eat. After I finish my food, I call Josh.

"Hi, how are you? When's your final exam?" I ask him.

"Hey, Mom, I'm good. My last exam is this afternoon." I feel his relief.

"Are you sure you'll be OK by yourself over the holidays?" I ask, concerned.

"Yeah, Dad is coming next week. As we discussed when you were here, I'm only off for two weeks, and then classes start again."

"I remember." *I still don't like the idea of him being alone for Christmas.*

"Thanks for the gift cards, Mom," Josh interjects.

"You're welcome. I love you."

"Love you too, Mom. Bye."

I'm happy to hear Josh's voice, but I'm still concerned. *God, please be with Josh and keep him safe for the next several weeks.*

Thankfully, the afternoon goes much quicker than the morning. I warm up my car and pull out of the parking lot to head to the airport. Audra calls just as I'm pulling up to the terminal. I spot her and pull over in front of the baggage claim.

"Hi, Mom," she sings out. I open the trunk and walk toward her.

"I'm so happy to see you." I give her a huge hug and help her get her luggage into the car. We talk nonstop for the half-hour ride home.

"What would you like for dinner?" I ask.

"Can we get sushi?"

"Perfect—you want to look online and order now?"

Audra orders several sushi rolls and miso soup. I'm happy to not have to cook.

Five minutes from home, I stop at the restaurant and Audra jumps out to get our order. Pulling into our driveway, sadness engulfs me. I will only have two of my children home for Christmas this year. Curt has a computer gaming competition, so he, like Josh, will not be home.

"What's wrong, Mom?" Audra asks, looking concerned.

"I was just thinking about Curt and Josh not being home for Christmas."

I wipe away my tears with my shirtsleeve. I start helping Audra bring in her suitcases.

"It will be a quiet Christmas, Mom," she offers as consolation to me.

"I've been blessed to have each of you home for Christmas all these years," I share with my daughter. "I feel sad and a little lost right now."

"Well, I'm here, Mom, and AJ is home too. We will make new memories."

I smile at my beautiful and wise daughter, who's comforting me.

It's Christmas morning, but I don't feel the same excitement that I normally do. I go through the motions of Christmas morning, starting with cooking my Christmas breakfast casserole and cinnamon rolls. Taking a moment to have my first cup of coffee, I put on my favorite Frank Sinatra Christmas CD. Grant helped me with all the Christmas stockings last night. I'm so grateful that Audra and AJ are home, but I'm still thinking about Curt being in South Korea with his new esports coaching position and Josh being in San Francisco alone.

I'm sad and a little emotional. *Who am I kidding? I'm feeling depressed and very emotional!*

I call Curt since his Christmas is almost over—it's ten o'clock at night in South Korea.

"Hi, Curt. Merry Christmas!"

"Merry Christmas, Mom."

"Thank you. It feels strange without you and Josh here," I share with him.

"I know, Mom. I had Christmas dinner with friends here," he tells me.

"I'm glad you had a good day. I love you. Sleep well."

"You too, Mom. Enjoy your Christmas Day. I love you," Curt says emphatically.

I hang up the phone and turn around to see Grant smiling at me.

"Good morning and Merry Christmas, beautiful," he says joyfully.

"Merry Christmas." Grant comes over and hugs me as tears stream down my face.

"Honey, what's wrong?" he asks me, concerned.

"I miss my sons not being here for Christmas."

Grant just holds me and kisses me. Between talking to Curt and feeling Grant's love, I start to feel a little better.

Audra and AJ come downstairs.

"Merry Christmas to both of you." I acknowledge my two youngest.

They come over to hug me too. I'm smiling now, feeling some Christmas joy returning.

"Let's eat." I take the breakfast casserole and cinnamon rolls out of the oven.

We eat casually around the kitchen island. I serve orange juice to the kids and mimosas to Grant and me. After breakfast, everyone helps clean up.

"Can I bring the presents into the living room, Mom?" AJ asks.

"Yes, and Audra, can you take the stockings down from the mantle?"

"Sure, Mom." She winks at me.

"Another mimosa?" Grant asks me with a smile.

"Yes—one more, please." I kiss him on the cheek.

Each of us finds a seat in the living room, and AJ passes out the presents. He gets the new phone that he wanted. It's Audra's turn to open her big gift. She unwraps the box only to find another box wrapped inside. And then another. And another.

Finally, she opens the small one at the bottom. It's a gift certificate to take scuba diving lessons.

"Thank you, Mom." Audra stands to give me a hug.

"You're welcome." I hug her tight.

There are lots of clothes and a robe for AJ, sweaters for Grant, and perfume for me. I gather all the wrapping paper, bows, and tags. I can see the living room floor again.

We watch *A Christmas Story* together. Even though we have all seen it several times, it still makes us laugh. After the movie, the kids go to their rooms to relax, and I get the ham ready to put in the oven. I pick up my phone to call Josh to wish him a merry Christmas. He answers on the third ring.

"Hi, Merry Christmas. How's your day going?" I say in one breath.

"It's good. I'm having dinner with friends tonight," Josh answers.

"Oh, I'm so glad to hear that. I miss you here. I love you." I choke back my tears.

"Love you too, Mom." I'm so relieved he's having dinner with friends. I sit down on the couch to rest for a while.

Good thing I set the timer; it wakes me up in time to check the ham. After I take out the ham, I start the mashed potatoes.

"Can I help you with dinner?" Grant asks me, returning from the garage where he had been reorganizing the shelves.

"Yes—can you set the table and carve the ham?"

"Of course I can." Grant kisses me on the cheek and starts his tasks.

I put the beans, mashed potatoes, and rolls on the table.

"Time for dinner!" I shout out, opening a bottle of wine.

"Cheers and Merry Christmas," Grant says after the blessing.

Everyone talks about their gifts and what they're doing over the holidays. Audra is going with her boyfriend to Georgia for a few days. AJ is going with his girlfriend to her grandparents' place at the beach. I smile, listening to their conversations.

The kids clear the table. Grant and I enjoy a few moments together on the back porch.

"Thank you for making today so special." Grant holds my hand.

"You're welcome. I appreciate you reminding me of all I have to be thankful for."

"And in one week, we will be husband and wife!" he exclaims.

"I can't wait. I love you." I look into Grant's eyes.

"I love you." He kisses me passionately.

After minutes of silence just holding hands, we both feel a chill. We collect our wine glasses and head in. Back inside, Grant takes out the pie and ice cream.

"Who wants pie? Who wants ice cream?" Grant asks everyone.

"Both for me!" AJ exclaims.

"Me too," says Audra.

"I will have just pie, thank you," I respond.

We gather once more around the table to enjoy our dessert. I love all the new Christmas memories, and I will always be thankful for the past memories too.

Thank you, God, for this wonderful Christmas.

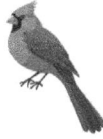

CHAPTER FIFTY-ONE

Friends for Christmas

Josh

I wake up freezing. I left the window open again last night. Jumping out of bed, I close it. Max finished his exams yesterday, and he went home to be with his family for Christmas. Both Mom and Dad offered to fly me home for the holidays, but I want to stay here.

I know spending time with my family is important, but I want to spend time with my new friends over the holidays.

In the shower, the scorching hot water warms me up. I'm really excited about the day. I dress in jeans and my green sweater. I grab a protein bar, my laptop, and my coat.

Once at school, I hurry to the lab to finish my project. It takes me forty-five minutes to finish it and submit it online. My last exam is in an hour, so I have time to go to the soda machine and get a drink. I don't normally drink soda, but I really want a Coke and need the caffeine to keep me awake during the exam.

Taking the exam, I know almost every answer. Computer programming is easy for me. It feels great to turn in my test.

I head down the stairs, into the lobby. Putting on my coat, I spot Laura coming out of the women's bathroom.

"Happy Friday," she announces to me and everyone in the lobby.

"Happy Friday," I reply, glad to see her.

"Are you done?" she asks me.

"Yes, I turned in my project this morning and just took my last exam."

"Lucky—I have one more to go. See you tonight at the party." Laura looks genuinely happy that I'm coming to the party.

"Yes, thank you again for inviting me." I smile at her and head out into the cold.

It's really cold today—the wind cuts right through me. Pulling out the hat Mom bought me, I realize that she's right: Winters in San Francisco can be quite cold. I climb the six blocks straight up to my apartment building. I wash my sheets and clean up my room. Cleaning out the fridge, I find a frozen meal and heat it up in the microwave.

Mom sent me several more gift cards. I especially like the movie and Visa gift cards. I go online to look for movies that are coming out for Christmas.

I have three hours until the party. I take another hot shower to warm up, and I shave too. Back in my room, I put on my clean jeans and my ugly Christmas sweater. I will take an Uber to and from the party. *Thank you, Mom, for another Uber gift card.*

There is one beer left in the refrigerator, a Bud Light. Not my favorite, but I'm happy for the alcohol to help me relax before I leave.

The Uber picks me up, and I head to Laura's apartment building. At the front door of the building, I can hear music coming from her apartment. I climb the stairs instead of taking the elevator. I knock loudly on the front door.

"Hi, Josh," Laura answers.

"Hey," I respond.

"Come on in," she says, waving me inside. I see several students that I know from school.

"Would you like a beer?" she offers. "Bud or PBR?"

"I will have a Bud, thank you," I respond.

"Help yourself to chips and dip and crackers and cheese." Laura smiles and turns away.

Before I can say anything else, she's answering the front door again. I find a group of kids I know and chat with them. About fifteen minutes later, Laura finds me.

"Would you like to smoke?" she asks me with a wink.

"Sure," I reply, following her to the porch where I see several more people I recognize.

Laura offers me a joint. We both sit down on a bench together.

"These are my roommates, Alexis, Ben, and Arnie." She gestures to each of them.

"Hi, I'm Josh," I say to the group. Ben and I have studied together. I didn't know he was Laura's roommate.

"Good to see you," Ben says, and then answers the question in my head. "I just moved in two weeks ago."

"Hey, I'm Arnie." He stands to shake my hand.

"Laura has talked about you. It's really great to meet you," Alexis adds.

We talk about school and where everyone is from. They love that I'm from the South, insisting that I can't be from there because I don't have a Southern accent. Both Alexis and Laura are from Southern California, Ben is from Colorado, and Arnie is from New York. I feel so comfortable smoking and talking with them.

I'm offered a myriad of drugs throughout the night. I stick to beer and weed. I'm feeling pretty good by the end of the night, or is it early morning?

Beer pong seems to be everyone's favorite game. I really suck at it, but I enjoy the conversations throughout the night. I don't get an Uber home until five in the morning.

I like hanging out with Laura and her roommates. I'm enjoying the start of my Christmas break.

I'm so tired, I don't even take off my ugly Christmas sweater. I smile, remembering I won the "ugliest sweater" contest.

With school out for two weeks, I'm back to sleeping in until noon or later. Laura sent me a message the day after the party, inviting me to Christmas dinner. I'm going to pick up a pecan pie on my way to her apartment. Mom calls just before I get to the apartment. I let her know that I'm spending Christmas with friends.

"Merry Christmas," I say to everyone as I enter the apartment.

"Hi, Josh. Come on in," Arnie says. "Would you like beer or wine?"

"Wine," I reply, surprising myself.

Dinner is really good. Laura made lasagna like my mom often makes for Christmas Eve. We laugh and drink throughout dinner. I bought a small gift for the gift exchange. I found a San Francisco bottle opener at the Ferry Building. I get two San Francisco–themed koozies in the exchange. Drinking and smoking gifts are very popular.

"Love the bottle opener. Thank you, Secret Santa." Alexis laughs out loud.

We play beer pong on Christmas night. I'm getting much better at this game. And I have fun singing Christmas songs while we play.

"C'mon, Josh, you must remember the words to 'Rudolph the Red-Nosed Reindeer,'" Ben challenges me.

"'All the other reindeer laughed,'" I sing.

"Close—'All the other reindeer used to laugh,'" Alexis corrects me.

"Drink, Josh," Laura says. I drink; I guess I don't remember many Christmas songs.

"Hey, Josh, you can crash on the couch," Ben offers.

"Thanks, man, I think I will." I say good night to everyone.

I don't sleep great on the couch, but I'm thankful for my new friends.

In the morning, Laura makes eggs and pancakes.

"Who wants eggs and who wants pancakes?" she asks everyone.

"Can I have both?" I ask with a wink.

"Of course, Josh," she responds, smiling.

We're happy to be on break; we play cards, watch movies, and play beer pong all day. Around nine o'clock that evening, I decide to get an Uber to head back to my place.

"Thanks for having me," I say to everyone.

"Great to have you, man," Ben responds for the group. "You're welcome anytime."

I smile as I walk out the front door.

Back at my place, I feel sad again. I'm realizing being alone makes me sad. *Will being sad lead me to feeling depressed again?*

Just then, the phone rings. It's Laura.

"Thank you again for having me for Christmas," I tell her.

"You're welcome, Josh. We have all been discussing something. One of Alexis's friends was going to move in, and now she's backed out. We would like you to move in."

"Wow, that would be great!" I'm happy she asked me. *It feels great to be included.*

"Ben and Arnie can help you move," Laura continues.

"I really appreciate that. Thank you, Laura, for everything. Good night."

I will move in three days before the New Year.

In bed, I look at some of the funny pictures from the party and Christmas.

I laugh out loud, remembering both nights. *At this moment, my heart feels full.*

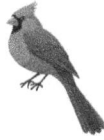

CHAPTER FIFTY-TWO

Much to Do

Maria

In three days, it will be New Year's Eve and our wedding day.

I'm excited to be marrying Grant. But I'm nervous about getting married again. Will we be happy together for the rest of our lives?

Audra helps me make a last-minute list of everything we need for the ceremony and the party afterward. The first stop today is the party store, to get the decorations.

"Since the cake is white fondant with a gold beaded trim, I would really like to add more decorations," I tell Audra as we walk into the store.

"We will find the perfect decorations, Mom."

In the party section, we find Roaring Twenties–themed plates, cups, and napkins. We get gold tablecloths, black-and-white platters to serve the food, and New Year's noisemakers.

"Mom, what about these black feathers to decorate the top of the cake with?" Audra shows me.

"Perfect, I'm so happy we're finding everything."

"The only thing left on our list is champagne glasses," Audra reminds me.

"It would be great to have real ones, but it's a New Year's Eve party, and the plastic ones will be just right."

Once we locate the glasses, we take our load to check out.

"Mom, other than the groceries and the drinks, we just need to order the balloons."

"Audra, thanks for all your help. It's going to be a wonderful celebration," I reply.

As we walk out of the store, I'm feeling sad again. *I want to honor Josh's decision to stay in California over the holidays. However, I'm disappointed that both he and Curt will be missing my wedding.*

Audra and I have talked about Grant and about us getting married. I've talked to AJ about it too. I could have discussed it more with Josh when I went to see him. And it's hard to gauge on the phone how Curt is feeling.

Maybe the kids are not excited at all about me getting remarried.

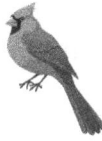

CHAPTER FIFTY-THREE

Happier Times

Josh

I spend the morning washing my clothes, blankets, and sheets. I start packing my stuff into my suitcase and several boxes. I throw away the leftover food that I didn't eat and clean out the fridge. Last, I take down my pictures and pack up my lamp, diffuser, and toiletries. Max found another guy from school who spends a lot of weekends with his family too. They will be good roommates. I leave Max the fan Mom bought for the room.

Just then, Arnie calls.

"Hi, Arnie—oh, you're here. Be right down." I hang up the phone and head downstairs.

I'm so excited to move in with them, yet I feel nervous too. *Why am I feeling nervous?*

"Hey, Josh, you ready to move?" Ben asks.

"Yes. Thank you again for inviting me to live with you guys."

It takes us less than ten minutes to get everything in the car. Thank goodness they are on the first floor. Another ten minutes later, and we have all my things in their apartment.

Ben and I will be rooming together. I don't have a dresser, so I hang up some of my clothes in the closet. I will use my suitcase as my dresser for now.

"Who wants pizza?" Alexis yells from the kitchen.

"Sounds great," Arnie and Ben say in unison.

"I will order two cheese and two pepperoni pizzas." Alexis places the order.

"Would you like a beer?" Ben asks me.

"Thank you," I reply, feeling so much gratitude. "For the beer and for having me stay here."

"You're welcome—we're glad to have you," Arnie says.

I chill on the outdoor porch with the guys until the pizza arrives. We help ourselves to several slices of pizza and more beer.

"So, Josh, tell us more about your family," Arnie asks me. He has thick black hair and a strong New York accent.

"I have three siblings. Curt, my older brother, is in South Korea working for a video game company. My sister, Audra, is studying marine biology at the University of Rhode Island. And my youngest brother, AJ, is a senior in high school in South Carolina."

"You're from Charleston, right?" Laura asks, joining us on the porch.

"Yeah, we moved there when I was five," I respond.

"What made you choose San Francisco?" Ben asks in his laid-back way.

"To be honest, last spring I traveled across the United States by bus, and I ended up here. I really like San Francisco. My aunt helped me find the school."

"That's cool that you could just pick up like that and try something new!" Alexis says.

"Thanks. It's been a bit of an adjustment, being on my own. I'm glad that I met all of you. It's been fun, and I enjoy being here." I look around at my new friends.

Laura smiles her beautiful smile and tucks her long blond hair behind her ears.

She takes hold of my hand. *I feel real joy being part of my new family.*

"The guys are in charge of the drinks for New Year's, and the girls are in charge of the food." Laura is the planner of the group.

Tomorrow, we will hit the liquor store and the local market for beer and wine. The girls will go to the grocery store to get party food and meals for the next three days. We watch the newest Spider-Man movie and call it a night. My new twin bed is better than the couch, but I still toss and turn all night. At least Ben doesn't snore.

The next morning, during breakfast, we make our grocery and alcohol lists. Ben is also making a list of what drugs to get. Weed is top of the list, but there are a few others.

I promise myself right then that I will stick to weed and beer. *I know that anything stronger can really mess me up.*

"You guys ready?" Ben asks.

"Yes, let me get my shoes." I go into the bedroom to grab my sneakers.

We go to the liquor store first. We get rum, vodka, tequila, and whiskey. Then, at the local mom-and-pop market, we pick up three cases of beer and eight bottles of wine—four red and four white. We drop all that off at the apartment and go to make the weed run. Ben knows a guy from school, and we're going to his place to get the weed. Apparently, he can also get us some cocaine. It really makes me nervous, but I go along with him.

Luckily, I get to stay in the car while Ben runs inside for the exchange. He's back in a few minutes, smiling from ear to ear.

"Thanks for keeping a lookout," Ben says as he gets in the car.

Wait! What? I was the lookout? I guess I did a good job. Good thing I didn't know that was my job. I don't want to have to do that again.

Back at the apartment, Ben stashes the drugs. After lunch, he offers me a hit.

"Thank you." *I do like to smoke weed.*

Everyone joins in throughout the afternoon. Ben opens a beer and offers one to me.

"Thanks," I say again.

The weather turns really cold and rainy. We're stuck inside for the next two days. Good thing we have enough to eat and drink. But now we're going to have to make another food and beer run before New Year's Eve.

"I made a new list," Laura offers to the group. "Alexis and I will restock the fridge."

"I have a gift card from my mom for Christmas. I could replace the beer."

"Thanks, Josh. And, Ben, can you get more weed for the party?"

"You know I can," Ben says, smiling.

The next morning, Alexis makes pancakes for all of us for breakfast.

"Wow, thank you." I smile at her. "I can definitely get used to this."

She smiles back and continues to make more pancakes for everyone. After breakfast, I borrow Laura's car to go to the mom-

and-pop store for more beer. I could walk, but I wouldn't be able to carry three cases of beer back. I pick a medley of cheap beer. When I get home, Ben's awake and about to head out to stock up on more weed. He helps me bring in the beer and get half of it into the fridge.

Thank God, this time Arnie is going with him to be the lookout.

"Bye, guys. See you in a bit." I finish putting the beer in the fridge.

I take a quick shower so the girls will have time to get ready too. It's a three-bedroom apartment, but there's only one bathroom. Luckily, my black jeans and green button-down shirt are clean. After I hang up my towel and put away my toothbrush and deodorant, I return to the kitchen.

"Josh, could you cut the cheese into cubes for the party?" Laura asks me.

"Sure, I can do that," I respond.

I pull out a knife, the cutting board, and the three types of cheese.

"Don't forget the colored toothpicks." She hands me the box.

"Wow, we're going to have a fancy party," I say, and she laughs. I cut the cheese quickly and stab each cube with a toothpick. The guys return, and I can tell they have been smoking weed on the drive home. I know I need to pace myself tonight.

All of my roommates like to party, and with my addictive tendencies I have to be very picky about what I take. *I will stick to pot again tonight.*

"Looking good," Ben says, pointing to my cheese platter.

"Thanks, man," I say to him. Then I ask Laura, "What else can I do to help?"

She tells me what to chop and stir. We have mini meatballs, chicken on a stick, small quiches, barbecue in the crockpot for barbecue sandwiches, and of course, my cheese platter. Alexis has made chocolate chip cookies and several types of dips for chips and dip.

"Ben, you're in charge of setting up the bar," Laura instructs him.

"I'm on it," Ben replies, pulling out all the liquor and wine.

Arnie's going to be the DJ for the night. Alexis serves each of us guys barbecue sandwiches and chips. She doesn't want us to eat all the appetizers before the guests arrive. I open my first beer to go with my barbecue sandwich. Our guests start arriving around half past eight.

"Hi, I'm Josh," I greet the first guest at the door.

"Hi, Josh, I'm Jessica. Laura's one of my good friends."

"C'mon in, it's nice to meet you. Can I get you a drink?"

"Yes, please. Can I get a gin and tonic?" she asks.

"Be right back." I smile at her.

"Gin and tonic," I tell Ben.

He mixes it up and hands it to me, smiling.

"She's Laura's friend." I motion toward the front door.

"I know, man," Ben says, laughing. I head back over to Jessica.

"Thank you," she says. "Oh, wow, this drink is strong!"

"That's how Ben likes his drinks," I explain.

"How long have you known Laura and the gang?" Jessica asks.

"About four weeks. We all go to school together."

"I go to Berkeley," she continues.

"Wow, do you like it?" I'm intrigued now—Berkeley students are very smart.

"I do, but it's a lot of hard work."

"What are you studying?" I ask her.

"Psychology. I want to be a counselor."

Oh. I'm not sure I should say I've been in therapy. This girl is beautiful and smart. We talk all night—she tells me about her younger brother and family who live in San Diego. I tell her all about my siblings, my parents, and growing up in Charleston.

"I have always wanted to go to Charleston." I just smile; everyone always says that.

Yes, it's a beautiful place, and it was nice growing up there, but I no longer understand the fascination. San Francisco has so much more to offer. I love the cable cars, the many different types of people, and the attractions and parks.

"I really like San Francisco. There's so much to do here." I share my thoughts.

"Yes, there is a lot to do and see." Jessica sips her drink.

"My mom was just here last month for a visit. She took me to Alcatraz, to Twin Peaks, and on a sunset cruise in the harbor."

"Wow, she had you on the go." Jessica smiles.

"Yes, I was a little irritated at first, but I really did have fun." I want to be honest.

"Do you get to see your family a lot?" Jessica asks me.

"Well, Mom was here in November, and Dad was here right before Christmas. I decided not to go home for Christmas since we had such a short break. But I feel bad now, because I'm missing Mom's wedding tonight."

"Oh wow, you didn't want to be there for that?" she asks in a concerned way.

"It's been weird with Mom, and I guess I wasn't ready for her to remarry even though my parents have been divorced for six years."

"I understand how you feel. My parents divorced two years ago. I've seen a therapist to share my feelings about it. Maybe that's why I want to be a counselor."

"I've been seeing a therapist too. I've had depression for a while," I share with her.

"Sorry you've had to experience that. How are you doing now?" she asks sincerely.

"I'm starting to feel better. The new medication has been helping, and I'm finally feeling like me." *I feel like I can tell her anything.*

"I'm so glad to hear you are starting to feel better." I can see by the genuine look on her face that she means that.

"Thank you," I respond.

"Oh, this is one of my favorite songs. Wanna dance?" she asks me.

"I'm not a great dancer, but I will give it go." I actually have fun dancing with her.

"It's almost midnight," Laura yells to everyone. She's been talking to every party guest throughout the night.

"Would you like some champagne?" I ask Jessica.

"Of course, I would love a glass." She smiles at me.

I walk over to Ben's elaborate champagne glass setup and take two glasses for us.

"Here you go," I say, handing Jessica a glass.

"Ten, nine, eight, seven, six, five, four, three, two, one. Happy New Year!" we all shout.

Jessica and I clink our glasses and drink our champagne, and I give her a quick kiss. We're both smiling.

"Happy New Year, Josh."

"Happy New Year!" I look at her, noticing her deep blue eyes.

We both have another glass of champagne on the porch. It's really cold outside, and I notice Jessica shivering.

"Would you like my coat?" I offer.

"Yes, please. Thank you," she answers. I hand her my coat I left on the chair.

We continue our conversation and enjoy each other's company beneath the stars.

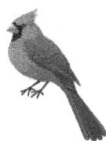

CHAPTER FIFTY-FOUR

New Year's Eve

Where's that higher love? ...
Until then I'll sing my song ...
I could light the night up
With my soul on fire
Let me feel that love come over me
—"Higher Love," Whitney Houston

Maria

It's New Year's Eve and our wedding day. Grant and I have invited our family and friends to celebrate with us. I chose a Roaring Twenties theme to ring in New Year 2020. Audra told me it was a silly idea, but even she's in the spirit after getting the party supplies.

"Good morning, beautiful." Grant greets me with my favorite French roast coffee.

"Good morning, and thank you," I respond with a kiss.

"I'm going to the store. Do you have the list?" he asks while getting his keys.

"I do; let me get it for you." I head to my desk to get the food and drink list.

After Grant leaves for the store, I make eggs, bacon, and pancakes. Audra comes out for breakfast when she smells the bacon.

"Morning, Audra."

"Good morning, Mom."

"Are you hungry?" I point to the cooked food.

"Yes—very," she responds. "No pancakes, though."

I serve us eggs and bacon. After cleaning up the breakfast dishes, we start on our list.

Audra helps me make a plan for the day. Listening to the great playlist Grant made for the party, I start moving furniture around, and Audra begins decorating.

Grant's picking up the cake too.

"Mom, it's great to see you smiling," Audra says.

"I feel great. Thank you for helping." I'm really excited for our celebration, yet I feel the sadness creep in, knowing my two older boys are not here.

"Sure, it's going to be a wonderful ceremony and party." Audra starts putting out the plates and napkins on the bar counter.

"I love the black, gold, and white balloons and how everything coordinates with the plates and napkins too." I look around the room.

"Are the gold tablecloths pressed, Mom?" Audra asks.

"Yes, they are upstairs in the laundry room."

"I'll get them and put them on all the tables." She heads upstairs.

While I'm washing all the serving trays, I hear Grant coming in the front door.

"I'm home," he announces to the whole house.

"Hi, I'll be right down to help bring in the cake."

He kisses me as we pass on the stairs, carrying the grocery bags.

I have a quick glimpse of Grant helping me in the future and making life fun.

We bring the cake up carefully, and Grant helps me extract it from the cake box. It's three layers of white fondant icing with a gold beaded trim around each round layer. The three layers are chocolate, vanilla, and red velvet.

"Audra, can you add the black feathers on top?" I ask her.

"Sure, Mom. I will, as soon as I cover this last table."

The cake looks great, and everything is coming together. It's time to start cooking. Grant is on chopping duty, and Audra helps me with the dips.

"Mom, I need a hammer to start hanging the lights," AJ says as he comes downstairs.

"It's in the garage," I tell him. "On the shelf to the right as you enter."

"After I put up the lights, I'm going over to Anna's house."

"Please be home by six o'clock this evening for the party."

"Will do." AJ grabs a bottle of water and heads to the garage.

"Thank you." I smile, knowing he's a teenage boy and would rather spend New Year's Eve with his girlfriend and his friends. *I'm thankful he will be at our wedding.*

After Grant chops up all the veggies for the veggie tray, he starts cutting all the cheeses. We prep all the cooking sheets with the fried shrimp and chicken satay. I will stick them in the oven just before the guests arrive.

"Honey, why don't you get ready first? Then I can shower after you," I offer to Grant.

"On my way." He kisses me again and makes me blush.

"What time is Kevin coming over?" I ask Audra.

"He said he'd be here around seven o'clock to help with last-minute stuff."

"That's very nice of him." I cover all the trays for the oven with aluminum foil.

"Mom, I'm going to go get ready now too." Audra heads to her room.

I sit down on the side porch even though it's chilly outside. It's so nice to reflect on the past year and set my intentions for the New Year. Grant joins me on the porch, showered and shaved. He hands me a glass of red wine.

"Cheers to our new life of adventure, love, and joy!" Grant toasts to us. "I love you."

"Cheers, I love you!" We clink our glasses.

"You clean up really nice." I admire how good he looks in his suit. "I better go get ready."

Getting out of the shower, I quickly dry my hair and put on my makeup.

I take another moment for myself. *I know marrying Grant is the best decision. But maybe I should have waited until Josh was feeling better and both of my older boys were home.*

I go to my closet and pull out my dress. Putting on my flapper dress of gold, black, and ivory makes me smile. I'm looking forward to celebrating with our loved ones. As I head downstairs, I start to feel festive.

"Wow, you look amazing," Grant says, walking toward me and taking me in his arms.

"Thank you." I blush again.

"You really do, Mom," Audra adds.

"You do too, Audra," I tell my beautiful daughter. She has on a black flapper dress covered in fringe.

I hear AJ get out of the shower and know he will be down shortly. Anna, his girlfriend, just arrived, wearing a gold dress and a beautiful gold headband.

"Well, let's get this party started!" Grant sets up his makeshift bar for the night.

As Audra helps me set out all the platters of food, the doorbell rings.

"I'll get it!" Audra shouts, running down the stairs. "Hi, Kevin."

They both come up into the kitchen.

"Thank you so much for having me." Kevin gives me a hug and shakes Grant's hand.

"Since you are staying in the guest room, would you like the first Prohibition-themed drink?" Grant asks him.

"Sure, that sounds great," Kevin agrees.

The guys bond over a Bee's Knees while I open more wine. Grant's music plays in the background, and I smile, acknowledging that we put our celebration together ourselves. More guests arrive, all dressed up in Roaring Twenties attire. Drinks are poured, and appetizers are added to small plates. Our dearest friends and family are here to celebrate our marriage and ring in the New Year.

Our friend and pastor, Steve, will marry us. Everyone gathers in the living room, and Pastor Steve begins the ceremony. He says a prayer, reads the Corinthians passage about love, and gives a brief sermon on the joy of marriage.

"Do you, Grant, take Maria to be your wife?" Pastor Steve asks Grant.

"I do," Grant responds.

"And Maria, do you take Grant to be your husband?" the pastor asks me.

"I do," I respond, looking into Grant's eyes.

"I now pronounce you husband and wife. Grant, you may kiss your bride."

Grant kisses me, and everyone cheers. Audra hugs me and then Grant. AJ gives me a big hug and shakes Grant's hand.

"Congratulations to Grant and Maria!" Janet toasts to us.

"Cheers!" everyone exclaims.

"Thank you all for being here to celebrate our marriage. Everyone help yourself to more food and drinks, and enjoy the night," Grant tells our guests as he turns up the music.

It's ten o'clock when Audra reminds me we should probably cut the cake. She's been taking pictures all night for me.

"Mom and Grant, hold the knife together for a picture," Audra instructs us.

Grant is nice and doesn't smear cake all over my face when he feeds me the first piece. We dance and laugh and play casino games. Grant found a small craps table and is teaching our guests to play. Audra is in charge of keeping the food trays full, and Grant has bequeathed his bartender duties to Kevin.

I help Kevin and Audra get all the champagne glasses filled for the toast, and everyone is given a flute just minutes before the countdown.

"Thank you for being here for our wedding and to ring in the New Year," Grant tells all of our guests.

"Ten, nine, eight, seven, six, five, four, three, two, one. Happy New Year!" everyone cheers. Grant kisses me.

Champagne flutes are refilled, and the party continues. An hour later, our guests start heading home. They each hug us goodbye and share more well-wishes.

Once everyone has left, Audra, Kevin, AJ, and Anna help us put the food away and clean up all the tables and counters.

Grant and I sit down on the couch to reminisce about our night. I'm pretty tired, but too excited for bed just yet. As my husband holds my hand, I know that he will always be there for me, and I will always be there for him.

"Good night, Mom." Audra stands up.

"Good night, Audra. Thank you for all your help today." I smile at her.

"You're welcome—it was a great celebration."

"I love you so much." I hug my wonderful daughter.

"I love you too, Mom."

I wake up on the first day of the new year married to a wonderful man who truly loves me. Our wedding celebration last night was filled with love and laughter.

I'm still feeling sad that Curt and Josh were not here. I hope they will always know how much I love them. And I hope all my kids know that I still care about Aaron as their father.

"Good morning, my beautiful wife." Grant comes to the side of the bed, gives me a kiss, and hands me a cup of coffee.

"Morning, my handsome husband." I kiss him and take the coffee cup.

"What would you like to do today?" he asks, interested in my response.

"Can we just wear our pajamas and watch some movies and maybe some football?" I ask him.

"That sounds perfect! Let me know when you want to have breakfast." Grant kisses me and heads downstairs. I could really get used to married life: coffee in bed, breakfast cooked to order, and spending all day together relaxing.

I enjoy my coffee and the first Bible reading and reflection in my new devotional—1 Thessalonians 5:16–18: "Rejoice always, pray continually, give thanks in all circumstances."

Thank you, God. I'm so thankful for joy in my life again.

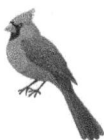

CHAPTER FIFTY-FIVE

Return to Normal

Josh

Classes begin again today. I've been sleeping much better during the break. *I really want to do well this semester. I know I'm smart, yet studying can be hard for me. I hope that when I experience sadness, I'm able to talk about it.*

Living in the new apartment, the school is much closer. I can roll out of bed, go to the bathroom, and get dressed. Five minutes later, I'm walking into class.

"Hi, Josh," Max greets me.

"Hi, Max, did your new roommate move in yet?" I ask him.

"Not yet, he moves in this week."

"No hard feelings, man?" I question him hesitantly.

"Not at all. I know I go home a lot," Max acknowledges.

"We can still study together, if that works for you," I offer.

"Sounds great." Max goes to take his seat.

Class starts, and I remember that programming this early in the morning is not fun. After class, I treat myself to a Starbucks breakfast sandwich and a hot tea. Luckily, I only have one lab this afternoon. When I get home later, the girls are back from school too.

"Hamburgers work for dinner tonight?" Laura asks.

"Yeah, sounds great. Can I help with anything?" I walk into the kitchen.

"Arnie is going to grill the burgers," Laura says, making hamburger patties. "Would you set the table?"

"Sure thing." I pull out the plates, silverware, and napkins.

Ben comes home very excited.

"Who wants to go to Mexico for spring break?" he asks us.

"Sure—where in Mexico?" I ask.

"Guadalajara," he responds.

"I'm in," Laura yells from the kitchen.

"Me too," Alexis says, coming into the living room.

"Arnie is in too. We can start looking at flights tonight," Ben continues.

"I will have to get a passport," I interject.

"You have time, but better start the process this week," Alexis explains.

"I'll look online and get my birth certificate from my mom." I can call Mom later.

"Arnie, the hamburger patties are ready," Laura adds to the conversation.

Arnie takes the burgers out on the porch to grill. Laura also made homemade macaroni and cheese to go with the burgers. Dinner is great, and we all talk nonstop about Mexico. Ben is in charge of flights, and Laura and Alexis will research hotels. After dinner, I step out on the porch to cover the grill and call Mom.

"Hi, Mom, Happy New Year. And congratulations!"

"Thank you, Josh. Happy New Year. How are you?" Mom asks.

"I'm good, and classes have started up again. Hey, my new roommates and I are planning a spring break trip to Guadalajara. Could you mail me my birth certificate?" I ask her.

"Oh, wow, Mexico! Isn't that part of Mexico a little dangerous?" Mom asks.

"No, Guadalajara is relatively safe," I share with her. "And flights are cheap."

"I can mail your birth certificate." I hear hesitation in Mom's voice.

"I will be safe, Mom." *I'm nervous about going to Mexico, but I really want to go.*

Later, Ben and I look at flights online; we find a great deal with JetBlue. We'll book the flights by tomorrow night. I send Dad a quick text to see if he can give me money as an early birthday gift. He says that's perfect since he had no idea what to get me this year. Five minutes later, I receive an email saying I have received money via Venmo. Dad has given me money for the flights and toward the room.

Thank you, Dad, I text to thank him.

I start the passport process online. I can mail everything in as soon as I get my birth certificate. Later, I will ask Mom to help me with money for the passport.

"Hey, Josh, you want to go with me this Saturday to get some shirts and shorts for the trip?" Ben asks me.

"Sure, I could definitely use some new shorts."

"This is going to be a fun trip," Laura chimes in.

"I've never been out of the country," I tell the group. I feel anxiety creep in.

"You are going to love it, Josh," Alexis shares. "We all travel a lot—it can be super addicting!"

I spend more time on my laptop, looking up fun things to do around Guadalajara.

I'm excited about my first trip out of the country and my first real spring break.

The anxiety must be because I've never flown out of the country.

It will be fun. And I will celebrate my twenty-first birthday in Mexico!

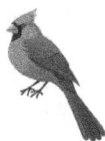

CHAPTER FIFTY-SIX

A Fresh Start

Maria

Every new year starts off with such promise. But historically, I have always hit some kind of challenge by mid-January. Having Josh so far away has been hard. I call Aaron to get his thoughts about Josh going on this trip.

"Happy New Year. How are you?" I ask Aaron.

"I'm good," he replies.

"That's good to hear. So, what are your thoughts about Josh going to Mexico?"

"I think it's great. He's in college, and he should be having fun."

"I agree. I want him to be a typical college student and have fun. But the idea of him going to Guadalajara scares me, even though I know it's safer than most areas of Mexico."

"Why don't you read about the city online?" Aaron always researches any new place.

"OK, I will do some more research." I feel a little better after talking to Aaron. And I have to trust Josh too. I pull out my laptop and google Guadalajara. It's a really pretty city with lots of history and Mexican culture. I will give Josh this gift for his birthday.

I send him a quick text. *Hi, how are you?*

Great, Mom. I'm excited about Mexico, he texts right back.

I'm going to send you $250 now, for your passport, and then $250 more right before you leave, for spending money.

Thank you so much, Mom.

You're welcome, Josh. I love you.

Love you too, Mom.

I'm happy and grateful that Josh has friends he's living with now and that they're all traveling together to Mexico. Josh is able to talk with his therapist via Skype, and he says he's still taking his medication.

God, please continue to give me peace, knowing you're with Josh.

I head upstairs to take a bubble bath.

"Hi, sweetheart." Grant greets me with a kiss. He worked late tonight.

"How was your day?" I ask.

"Long. I missed you." He kisses me again. "Did you have a good day?" he asks me sincerely.

"A little stressful at work, and I'm a little worried about Josh."

"Can I bring you a glass of red wine?" Grant offers.

"Yes, please, that would be great." I relax.

I start the hot water and pour in extra bubble bath. Grant comes back with my wine and another kiss. Once the water fills the tub and the bubbles are higher, I slip into the hot water.

My stress is washed away by the hot, soapy water, but more so by my trust in God. Josh is a young man now, and he needs to learn how to navigate the world with his mental challenges.

I will have to let go and stop treating him like a little boy. I can ask him occasionally how he is, and I need to trust that he will let me know if he's feeling bad. I'm so proud of him for making a move on his own to go to school in California. I have to trust that he can make big decisions on his own now.

Closing my eyes, I listen to Carla Bruni, my favorite French singer, on Alexa.

After my bath, I put on my silk pajamas and crawl into bed. I journal my intentions for the new year. I'm more at peace now. Sleep catches up with me. The last thing I remember is Grant kissing my forehead and turning off my bedside lamp.

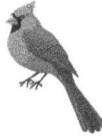

CHAPTER FIFTY-SEVEN

Tropical Escape

Josh

We leave for Mexico today. I've not felt this happy in such a long time. All of us were up early, adding the last few things to our suitcases and getting breakfast. Alexis has called a van shuttle company to take us to the airport. Being so early, there is little traffic. We arrive at the airport in plenty of time, and the line moves quickly as we go through airport security.

Once at our gate, we have twenty minutes before we board our eight o'clock flight. I go in search of water and some snacks.

We board and find our seats on the plane. *I feel anxious about flying to another country.* I breathe in and out several times. *Hopefully I can sleep on the plane.*

Opening my eyes, I can see the blue water below as the plane descends. I slept the whole flight! We take a taxi from the airport to our hotel. Check-in is at three o'clock, but they let us check in thirty minutes early. The guys have one room, and the girls have another.

"Let's meet back in the lobby in fifteen minutes to go check out the town," Laura states.

Arnie, Ben, and I just dump our suitcases on our beds. I decide to carry my passport in my front pocket along with my phone, cash, and credit card. The girls are in the lobby when we get off the elevator.

"Where to first?" Alexis asks.

"The local cantina," Ben quickly responds.

"Great idea," Arnie agrees.

The town has many old buildings, with modern stores and restaurants in between. We find the perfect bar with margarita and beer drink specials. I decide that my first drink will be a Mexican beer. With drinks in hand, we all yell, "Cheers!" and clink our glasses together. Two drinks later, we order several plates of food to share. Looking around at my friends, I see that everyone looks as happy as I feel.

I close my eyes to really feel this amazing moment with my friends.

We walk around the rest of the afternoon, stopping at booths in the market. I love watching the girls hold up Mexican shirts, dresses, and trinkets. Ben is restless—I know he would rather be drinking in a local bar. Arnie and I are both happy just taking in the authentic culture all around us. We end up at another restaurant and bar on the water. This time, we indulge in two rounds of margaritas. I'm definitely feeling the alcohol now.

It's obvious we're American, but we don't care that we stand out.

"Who's ready to head back to the hotel?" Alexis asks. "We can do it all again tomorrow."

The sun set about ninety minutes ago, and we all agree it's time to call it a day.

Taking a cab, we're back to the hotel in five minutes and in our beds minutes after that.

I hear Arnie start to snore. *Oh, no, will I be able to fall asleep?*

I feel grateful that I said yes to going to Mexico with my friends. *And it feels great to leave depression behind.*

I guess I did fall right to sleep. The next thing I see is the sun coming through the blinds, waking me up. Both Ben and Arnie are still sleeping, so I hop in the shower. The water is super hot, and I dance around in the shower, trying to rinse all the soap off of my body. After putting on one of my fun Hawaiian shirts and some shorts, I slip out the door and head to the lobby.

Laura is there; she has two cups of coffee and what looks like donuts.

"Hi, good morning," she sings out. "Happy twenty-first birthday!"

"Good morning," I say back. "Thank you!"

"Please have the other cup of coffee and a churro," she offers.

"Thank you so much." The churro is one of the best things I have ever tasted. I love the sweetness and the way it melts in my mouth.

"You want to take a walk on the beach before the others get up?" Laura asks.

"Yeah, I'm up for a walk. Thank you again for breakfast."

It's hot outside already at 8:00 a.m.

The sky is deep blue with "happy clouds"—that's what I like to call the white fluffy ones. The sand here is much coarser than the sand on the beaches in South Carolina. It feels strange between my toes. We wade into the ocean. The water is so clear we can see the bottom, and it's much cooler than I thought it would be.

We walk along the beach for a while and practice our Spanish.

"*Una cerveza, por favor?*" I ask Laura.

That's my favorite Spanish phrase—"One beer, please."

We see several families carrying toddlers and beach gear to spend the day at the beach. Turning around to head back, Laura yells, "Last one back is a rotten egg!"

I immediately think of Carrie. I wonder if she's hanging out with another guy. By the time I start running, Laura is way ahead of me. She stops and turns around.

"You coming?" she challenges me.

I run faster and almost run into her. Laughing, she starts running again. We run together to the water.

"Guess I need to start exercising more," I say, laughing with her.

When we get back to the hotel, everyone's in the lobby.

"Happy birthday, Josh!" they all sing out together.

"Thank you," I respond, blushing.

"Where were you two?" Alexis asks.

"We took a run on the beach," Laura explains.

"Cool," Ben responds.

"So, what are the plans for today?" Arnie asks.

"We can rent ATVs and ride on the north beach," Ben offers.

"That's a great idea," Alexis chimes in.

Getting directions from the hotel concierge, we head out toward our destination. Everyone gets their own ATV. Laura is afraid to ride by herself, so I offer for her to ride shotgun with me.

"Thank you, Josh."

"Sure, we'll have a blast." I wink at her.

We start in a line, following Ben. Once we reach the farthest point of the north beach, we all take off in different directions. The view of the ocean is amazing as we travel on the gravel road right along the water. It's exhilarating driving with the wind whipping all around us. Laura and I get off the ATV to explore the rockier coast by foot.

"You want to drive now?" I hand her the keys.

"Yes, I would like to." She hops on, and I climb on behind her. She's a natural—I'm not sure why she didn't want her own ATV. I'm definitely not complaining; I really enjoy spending time with her.

"You might want to slow down a little," I yell over the engine.

She lets off the gas a little, but we're still going really fast.

We beat everyone back.

"Wow, that was a lot of fun!" Laura exclaims.

"Yeah, you're a pro," I tell her.

We return the ATVs and helmets. It's another five minutes before the others show up.

"Laura, you can really ride," Ben acknowledges.

"Thanks, we'll have to do that again."

"All right, let's go find the closest cantina. I'm really thirsty," Arnie says.

Luckily for us, there are several cantinas within walking distance. The first one has outdoor seating and giant margaritas. We order the giant margarita to share. It's so huge that we each get two regular-sized margaritas out of it.

"CNN was on the television in the hotel lobby. Have any of you seen the news lately?" Alexis asks.

We all shake our heads. We have disconnected from social media on our phones.

"Apparently, there's a virus that's spreading really fast, and many countries are requiring people to stay home."

"What's the United States doing?" Arnie asks.

"Not sure, but we may want to call the airlines tomorrow," Alexis says.

"Why would we do that?" Ben asks.

"Just to be sure we can fly back to the US," Alexis continues. "I will call the airlines in the morning. But tonight, we're going to have fun celebrating Josh's birthday."

"OK, birthday boy, you get the first shot," Laura says with a tequila shot in hand.

They all yell, "Happy twenty-first birthday, Josh!"

I drink the shot solo.

"Wait, that's no fun," Ben shouts. "I'll get the next round of shots for all of us."

Several shots later, we're all feeling tipsy.

"Time to find food," Alexis insists.

We follow her to the restaurant down the street. Sharing appetizers, quesadillas, and tacos, we eat until we're stuffed.

"OK, let's all get changed so we can take Josh out dancing for his birthday." Laura has talked about dancing in Mexico for weeks. *I want to tell her I really can't dance.* She leads us back to the hotel, talking about the best places to go dancing.

After my shower, I put on my favorite Hawaiian shirt and tan shorts. The food helped, but I still have a good buzz going. I purchase bottled water at the front desk and chug the whole liter. I know I'll have to drink as much water as I can throughout the night. The birthday drinks will be plentiful, and I have to stay well-hydrated.

"Party time!" Laura yells as she and Alexis get out of the elevator.

"*Sí*," we all say in unison.

Outside the hotel, we pile into a taxi. The driver drops us off downtown where the nightclubs line both sides of the street.

"You ready, Josh?" Laura asks me.

"Ready as I'll ever be," I reply, smiling.

"First round is on me," Arnie says, and he disappears into the crowd.

I'm shocked at how packed the club is at nine in the evening. Laura's smiling at me as I survey the room. Arnie returns with more tequila shots.

"Happy birthday to Josh!" everyone cheers again.

We drink several more shots, and then I switch to beer.

"OK, birthday boy, time to dance," Laura shouts above the music.

Grabbing my hand, she pulls me out onto the dance floor. I give it my best, and we dance a few songs together.

"You're a good dancer," Laura says, encouraging me.

"Thank you," I say, feeling very embarrassed.

Back at the table, we laugh and drink and watch the crowd. I switch to bottled water and drink as much as I can before Ben offers me my next beer.

Laura smiles and blows me a kiss. I really like Laura, but our friendship is more important to me.

Having friends that understand me is awesome. This is one of the best birthdays ever!

"Time to go—the taxi is here." Ben directs us outside.

With everyone recalling the day, the ride home is the perfect ending to my birthday.

"Thank you, everyone, for such a wonderful birthday."

"It was so much fun celebrating with you," Alexis tells me.

"You're welcome, Josh." Laura smiles.

"Good night, Laura. Good night, Alexis," I say as we get off on our floor.

"Thanks again, guys," I say back in our room.

"Anytime, man. Today was a great day," Arnie replies.

"Sure thing, it was a blast," Ben adds.

In the bathroom, I brush my teeth and smile at my reflection. Laura does make me happy.

Why am I thinking of Carrie again? We're not together; I have no reason to feel guilty.

I guess I just miss her.

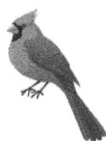

CHAPTER FIFTY-EIGHT
Motherly Vigil

Maria

I took a few days off to fly to Rhode Island and see Audra. She's not been feeling herself—she gets dizzy a lot, experiencing many déjà vu moments, and she's forgetting things. When she came home at Christmas, I took her to see a primary care doctor and a neurologist. As she went back to college in January, we scheduled an appointment with a neurologist at Massachusetts General Hospital in Boston.

I fly into Boston and rent a car to drive to pick Audra up. After two hours of driving, I finally pull into the drive behind her house on campus.

"Hi, sweetheart." I wave to Audra.

"Hi, Mom," she says, walking toward me.

I give her a huge hug.

"Wanna see my room?" Audra asks.

"Of course I do." I follow her up the back stairs.

"Not much to see, but it's cozy." Audra picks up her backpack.

"It's college—most rooms are small," I respond.

"I just need to pack my computer into my backpack."

"OK, let me carry your overnight bag," I offer.

We put Audra's bags in the car and head back toward Boston. We're staying at a Marriott close to the hospital. She has an MRI scheduled tomorrow morning and an EEG scheduled the morning after. Being able to walk to the hospital in the morning will save time.

We sing country songs the whole ride. I learn a few Dustin Lynch songs since we're seeing him tomorrow night at the House of Blues. It's my birthday present from Grant. Audra and I are both looking forward to the concert.

After checking in, we go to the local Whole Foods to pick up dinner, water, and snacks. In our hotel room, we talk and laugh and watch Audra's favorite teen movie, *Ten Things I Hate About You*. I want us to enjoy tonight. Once Audra has her tests results back, we can discuss her fears and concerns.

I am worried about her physical and emotional health. I know this is different from what Josh is going through. And yet I feel the same fear—will my kids be OK?

I want both Audra and Josh to be healthy.

Both of us head to bed early so we can get up by six in the morning.

The morning comes way too fast. Rushing around the hotel room, we get dressed, and I make coffee. Audra's MRI is scheduled for today.

"You nervous about this test?" I ask my daughter.

"No, not really. I just want to get it over with."

"OK, let's go. Hopefully they can get you in and out." I push the elevator button.

Audra has the first appointment of the day, and they take her right back. I read my devotional and pray while she's getting her MRI.

Today's scripture is Jeremiah 29:11: "For I know the plans I have for you ... plans to prosper you and not to harm you, plans to give you hope and a future." I will share the verse with Audra and her brothers—and especially with Josh, to encourage him.

Audra is done in half an hour. We're both happy that we have the whole day ahead of us.

"Starbucks for breakfast?" I suggest to her.

"Yeah, that sounds great, Mom."

It's really cold in Boston on March 1st. Luckily, Starbucks is right across the street.

"What else would you like to do today?" I ask.

"Can we go to the aquarium?" Audra inquires with a wink.

"Yes, that's a great idea!"

We take the rental car back and then get an Uber to the aquarium. I'm excited to go to the New England Aquarium. Looking at Audra's face, I can see she's excited too. We go right to the top of the fish tank that's several floors tall. It is filled with sea turtles and numerous fish of every species. Audra asks one of the aquarium guides several questions about the turtles. My young marine biologist is in her element. She knows as much as the guide who has been there many years.

After exploring the whole aquarium and watching the penguins, we decide it's time to head back to the hotel. We rest by watching *Pretty Woman* on cable. We take turns showering to get ready for dinner and the concert.

I select an Uber pickup, and we wait in the lobby. The Uber driver picks us up five minutes later and takes us right to the front entrance of the House of Blues. Grant has reserved a table for dinner and VIP access to the concert. Once we are seated, the server points out her favorites on the menu and tonight's specials. I have filet mignon, and Audra has a delicious pasta dish. With dinner, I have a glass of red wine to celebrate my birthday.

"Happy birthday, Mom." Audra toasts me with her iced tea.

"Thank you. I'm so happy to be spending my birthday with you."

After dinner, we go to find our seats. Grant also got us great seats for the concert.

Thank you for the great seats. I love you. I send him a quick text.

You're so welcome. Enjoy the concert. I love you, Grant responds.

Audra and I don't know the opening act, but his country songs are really good. When Dustin Lynch comes out, we dance and sing along.

We leave right after the concert since we have an early morning again. Audra has to stay up and can only sleep a few hours before her EEG in the morning. I decide it's best for me to go right to bed.

The morning comes way too early again. We walk to the hospital and head to the seventh floor. It's Monday morning, and the office is very busy. They take Audra back, and the EEG takes much longer than the MRI. The EEG will diagnose seizure disorders.

God, please be with Audra.

An hour and a half later, Audra comes back out to the waiting room.

"Hi, sweetheart. How did it go?" I ask her.

"Mom, it went OK. Can we go back to the hotel?"

"Sure," I respond, knowing she's tired. At least we have some time together today.

We both shower, and Audra packs up her bags.

"Would it be OK if you took me to the train station this morning?" she asks.

"Oh, I thought we were going to spend the day together. But I can take you to the train station this afternoon."

"If I get on the eleven o'clock train, I can make my class this afternoon."

"Of course," I say, defeated. "Can I at least buy you breakfast?"

"Sure, that would be great," Audra answers.

We get breakfast at the hotel to save time.

"Audra, are you scared about the results of your test?" I ask my daughter while we're waiting for our food.

"Yeah, I'm a little scared. I don't want to think about the results all day. And I'm really tired. If I head back now, I can go to class and be caught up."

I'm sad, but I respect my daughter's wishes.

After we eat, we're in another Uber, heading to the train station. I wait with Audra until they call for her train.

"I love you, and I'm so glad I got to see you and spend time together," I say to her.

"Me too, Mom. I love you." I can see that Audra is thankful for my help.

We hug, and she turns to get on her train.

I watch her go with tears in my eyes.

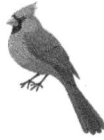

CHAPTER FIFTY-NINE

A Beach in Mexico

Josh

The next morning, we all stay in bed until noon to sleep off the effects of the alcohol from yesterday. I actually feel OK; drinking all that water helped me. We meet the girls in the lobby and head out together in search of food.

"How about spicy Mexican food and more beer?" Arnie asks.

"Perfect—I'm really hungry," I answer.

At the restaurant, several TVs are showing the same news station.

"What are they talking about?" Ben asks.

"Apparently, this worldwide virus is spreading fast. It's similar to the flu but worse. It's highly contagious, and people are dying from it," Alexis explains. "I've been following the NBC news app on my phone."

"Many countries are shutting down businesses and telling people to stay home," Arnie adds.

"What about the United States and Mexico?" I ask.

"Larger cities are starting to close down businesses in the US," Alexis tells me.

"Apparently, there are no shutdowns here in Mexico," Arnie adds.

"Will we be able to fly back to California in a few days?" Laura asks.

"I've been checking the airline's website, and there haven't been any cancellations yet." Alexis is watching out for all of us.

"Well, I say we continue to enjoy our spring break since we're here in sunny Mexico." Ben lifts his glass.

"Cheers," we all say in unison and order more beer.

"Hair of the dog is a silly saying, but it's so true," Arnie says, changing the conversation.

"Yeah, I'm feeling better after drinking a couple of Coronas." I push my bottles to the middle of the table. I'm not sure how I feel about the pandemic. *All I know is this time with my friends is so special to me, and I don't want it interrupted by some virus.*

"You know what's weird, guys? That's what they are calling it—the 'corona' virus. It's the scientific name shortened," Alexis explains.

"Alexis, I thought we were changing the conversation?" Laura interjects.

"Yes, we are, but it's funny because we're here in Mexico drinking a lot of Corona beer," Ben says, laughing.

"I say we hit the beach today and rent surfboards and just chill." Laura loves to plan.

"That sounds perfect, Laura," Arnie agrees. "Josh and I can get the beer and a cooler."

"I can find a good place to rent surfboards," Ben adds.

"Alexis and I will get towels, snacks, and sunscreen." Laura smiles at me.

We pay our bill and set out to accomplish our tasks, agreeing to meet back at the hotel. One thing that I love is that we're all efficient with our time. Half an hour later, we all have our bathing suits on and our supplies in hand.

"OK, let's do this," Ben says, leading us to the beach.

It's a quarter mile to the beach. The guys take turns carrying the surfboards. It's a beautiful day, with blue skies, and the water is turquoise. We pick our spot and set up our towels.

We drink Corona, swim, laugh, play Frisbee, and just relax. I even attempt surfing, although Arnie and Ben are much better at it. My favorite part of the day is talking with Laura about school and life. She's seen me down before and shared with me that she gets depressed sometimes too. *I love that she just accepts me as I am—that's a real friend.*

"Josh, where did you go? You were daydreaming," Laura teases.

"I was just thinking that you're always there for me," I respond. "You accept me."

Laura takes my hand, and we just sit in silence, watching the sunset.

For the first time, I feel a peace wash over me. I breathe in the salt air. Part of my emotional pain just drifts away. I can allow healing for my body and my mind.

When the sun finally sets, we pack up our beach gear. Arnie and Ben took the surfboards back earlier, so all we have is an empty cooler, sunscreen, Frisbees, and towels. We spot a local sandwich shop and get sandwiches and soft drinks for dinner. Still recovering from yesterday and from the sun and activity today, we're all really tired. We agree to call it an early night and head back to the hotel.

"Good night. See you guys in the morning," Alexis sings out.

"Good night," the guys say in return.

I shower and hang up my wet bathing suit and T-shirt. Crawling into bed, I recall another amazing day in Mexico.

I'm truly thankful for this great group of fun and caring friends.

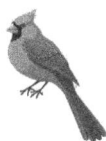

CHAPTER SIXTY

Uncertain Return

Maria

I'm heading to the airport to fly home to Charleston. Thank goodness, I get through security quickly. I notice that many people are wearing masks. I gravitate away from people, my intuition telling me to keep to myself. At the gate, the news on the television is about the worldwide pandemic. The airlines are talking about grounding flights.

"Is this flight still departing?" I ask the attendant at the desk.

"Yes, ma'am," the attendant answers.

"Thank you," I respond, and then return to my seat.

I send a quick text to Grant. *I'm boarding soon. I love you.*

I can't wait to see you. I love you, he quickly responds.

They start calling first and business class—Grant bumped me up to priority seating. I'm thankful to have a little more room. More and more people board the plane with masks on. I still have my scarf on since it was freezing when I left the hotel this morning. I wrap it tighter around my neck, covering my mouth too.

I remember the plane taking off; however, I must have slept through the whole flight. Waking up disoriented, it takes me a moment to realize that we're landing soon.

Hi, we just landed. I will meet you at baggage claim, I text Grant as we taxi to the gate.

OK, I'm here. See you soon, he texts me back.

Once I get off the plane, I head to baggage claim. Grant is there waiting for me, and he scoops me up in a huge hug and kisses me.

"Hi, beautiful. I'm glad you are home."

"I'm happy to be home." I kiss him again.

We walk to Grant's car. He puts my bags in the trunk and then holds the passenger door open for me. I tell him all about the aquarium, the concert, and spending time with Audra. I give him the details about Audra's appointments and tell him about feeling sad that she wanted to go back to school early. I talk nonstop all the way home. Grant just nods and listens.

"I'm just glad you're home, with everything going on in the world," he says.

"Yeah, I just saw the news today about the pandemic," I respond. "Have you heard about any airlines cancelling flights?

"I have not, no. I'm thankful you were able to fly home." Grant squeezes my hand.

"I hope they don't cancel flights before the weekend. Josh is flying back to California from Mexico on Saturday."

"Oh, that's right. He and his friends are still there on spring break."

"I will reach out to him tomorrow, see if he's heard about what's going on, and find out about his return flight," I say, worried about Josh getting back to California or getting sick.

"Are you hungry?" Grant asks me.

"I'm very hungry," I respond.

"Let's stop at the barbecue place since it's close to home," he suggests.

"Perfect. Can we get beer too?" I love a good beer with barbecue.

"Of course. I have been wanting to try a new IPA."

We order our favorite barbecue platter to share and our beer.

"Thank you for dinner and for picking me up at the airport."

"Anytime. You're welcome." Grant winks at me.

We pay the check, and as we're leaving, the news catches my attention: Hundreds have died in Italy, and the country is now in quarantine.

"Wow, it's really serious." I look to Grant.

"Yeah, people have been talking about it at work," he says.

"Speaking about work, I really don't want to go back tomorrow."

"Me either," Grant says with a laugh.

"Will we be able to go to the open house this weekend?" I ask. "We have three months to find a new place."

"Of course. I can call the real estate agent tomorrow," Grant offers.

On the drive home, I feel panic sink in. Then I feel fear for my kids, for my family and friends, and for Grant and me. This pandemic is serious.

At home, Grant helps me carry in my suitcase. I unpack and put on my comfortable yoga pants and sweatshirt. We decide to watch a movie and just relax together; I don't want to watch any more news. I cuddle up next to Grant and drift off to sleep.

Grant gently wakes me when the movie is over.

"You must have loved this movie," he says, teasing me.

"Sorry. I didn't sleep well at the hotel."

"You feeling all right?" Grant looks concerned.

"Yes, I'm just really tired," I reply.

"Well, off to bed for you." He kisses me on the cheek.

"Yes—a good night's sleep, and I'll feel much better tomorrow. I love you. Good night."

"Night, beautiful. I love you. I will be up soon."

I put on my pajamas and get into bed. I journal a little about my trip to see Audra, and I write my concerns about Josh being in a foreign country. I put my journal down and begin praying.

God, please protect my sons, Josh, AJ, and Curt, my daughter, Audra, Grant and me, and our family and friends from this contagious virus.

I close my eyes and fall right to sleep.

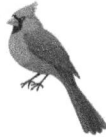

CHAPTER SIXTY-ONE

Real Fear

I can't stand to fly ...
I'm just out to find
The better part of me ...
And it's not easy to be me ...
Even heroes have the right to bleed
—"Superman," Five for Fighting

Josh

Wow, it's almost noon when I wake up. The guys are still in bed too. I put on a clean T-shirt and shorts. I grab the room key and exit the room. Both Alexis and Laura are sitting in the lobby.

"Hi, good morning, sleepyhead," Laura says.

"Good morning," I return.

"Are you hungry? Alexis and I were just about to go in search of food."

"Yeah, sounds good." My stomach grumbles just then.

We venture out of the hotel, hoping to find a place that's still serving breakfast. Luckily, just down the street, we find a mom-and-pop restaurant that serves breakfast all day. Both Alexis and Laura order omelets, and I order *huevos rancheros* with extra hot sauce. Our food comes quickly. I have to keep telling myself to slow down, but I'm so hungry. Two cups of coffee and a cinnamon churro complete my meal. I'm stuffed, but very happy.

"So what's the plan for today?" Alexis asks.

"Can we just explore the town and do a little shopping?" Laura looks to me for my input.

"Sounds good to me—we still have lots to see here." I'm not a fan of shopping, but I want to look around.

We bring the guys churros and bottled water. They're still asleep, so I leave the snacks in the room for them. The girls and I walk around the city of Guadalajara; the shops are filled with many authentic Mexican items.

"Here, Josh." Laura hands me a sombrero. I put it on, and the girls both laugh.

"Yes, you definitely need one of those." Alexis chuckles.

"Uh, I don't think so," I say, laughing too.

Alexis and Laura both purchase woven baskets and silver jewelry. I don't get anything; I just enjoy their company. Several hours later, we decide it's time to get a drink. We backtrack toward the hotel and go to our favorite bar. Ben and Arnie are already a beer ahead of us.

"Hi, guys. Are you both well rested?" Alexis asks.

"Yes—vacation is for fun and rest," Ben returns, smiling.

"Thank you for the churros and water," Arnie chimes in.

"You're so welcome," Laura responds.

"What did you guys do today?" Ben asks us.

"We walked around Guadalajara and did some shopping," Alexis shares.

"Whatcha get me?" Arnie asks.

"We couldn't find the right sombrero for you, although Josh looked quite handsome in the one he tried on," Laura says, smiling at me.

"So, any word about the flight?" Arnie asks.

"Still scheduled to leave at noon on Saturday," Alexis responds.

"OK, well, today is Thursday, so we have two more nights to party," Ben announces to the whole bar.

"Time for shots, then," I say, smiling.

"Tequila with Corona chasers?" Ben offers, heading to the bar.

After two rounds, we start talking about dinner.

"I love traditional Mexican food, but I would really like seafood," Alexis adds.

"Yeah, that sounds good." Arnie starts looking up seafood restaurants on his phone.

"We can go to the town of Tequila," Ben suggests.

We all agree that would be perfect. It's a thirty-minute train ride, and the restaurant Arnie picked is a few blocks from the train station. It's a family-style restaurant, and we share fish, shrimp, and *birria*, a spicy goat stew with vegetables. We eat, drink, and laugh.

Tequila is a very cultural and historical town. But Ben finds a poolside tequila-themed bar at Hotel Villa Tequila. It's definitely a popular hot spot for our crowd. I never knew there were so many different kinds of tequila. Ben is determined to try them all.

We have just been smoking pot this week. One of the clerks at the hotel says he has a friend in town who can get us cocaine. *I'm really nervous about getting drugs in a foreign country. I didn't like Ben getting drugs in California.*

While Arnie and the girls are getting ice cream, Ben and I meet this "amigo" at a dive bar down the street. We make the exchange and head to the train station to meet the others.

Arnie hands us our tickets. We wait thirty minutes for the next train.

"Thank you, Arnie. That was a lot of fun," Alexis says.

Walking back from the train station in Guadalajara, I notice the same guy from the exchange in Tequila standing outside our hotel with two of his friends. Because we had to wait for the train, they got here faster in their van.

"Hey, you," the one guy says to Ben. "My friend says you stole from him."

"Think you may have it wrong—we paid for it," Ben replies confidently.

"You definitely stole from us," the other guy states.

He hits Ben in the stomach, and my friend falls to the ground. I go to help him up, and the guy shoves me. I feel something poking in my side. *Gun.*

"Get in the van!" the man yells at me.

The second guy produces a gun too. I stumble toward the van. I see Ben getting up as they shove me in the back of the vehicle.

"No!" I hear him scream.

The bigger guy tightly binds my hands and mouth with black handkerchiefs.

They take my wallet and my phone. As they talk, I catch bits and pieces. I should have paid more attention in Spanish class.

"OK, asshole, here's what's going to happen. You will return the cocaine you stole, and we'll take all the money you have."

Why do they think I have the drugs?

I think of my family. *Mom. Dad.*

No. I'm going to die!

We drive and drive, and I have no idea where we are. I close my eyes and say a prayer silently. *Be strong and courageous.* I remember this scripture from Joshua on a card from Mom. I am scared. *They're going to shoot me. And leave me to die. God, save me.*

The men continue talking in Spanish. The smaller guy comes over to me. He raises his gun.

I finally want to live, and these thugs are going to kill me.

I feel sick to my stomach. I close my eyes.

All of a sudden, the van stops.

"Get out!" the man screams.

He pushes open the back door. I jump out of the van.

He throws my empty wallet and phone at me.

And they speed away.

I fall to the ground.

Breathe, I remind myself.

My hands and mouth are still bound.

I open my eyes and see my phone is somehow not broken. My open wallet is empty, but I hid my passport in our room. I look up to see that I'm at the end of a street near our hotel.

"Thank you, God," I whisper into the night. I start shaking.

They could have killed me. Miraculously, I'm still alive.

"Oh my god!" Laura yells. She and Alexis are coming out of the hotel.

They both run toward me.

"What happened?" Alexis asks as she and Laura untie the handkerchiefs.

Tears start to stream down my face. Laura hugs me hard. She sits down beside me, holding my hand. I gather my courage to tell them what happened.

"They shoved me into the van and tied me up. Then they just drove. They said we stole from them. They took all my cash. They threw my wallet and my phone."

I pause and try to control my tears.

"I'm so thankful you're alive!" Laura exclaims, hugging me tighter. "We called the cops when they took you. The cops came, and Ben freaked out and ran from them."

"Well, they just can't get away with this," Alexis says as she begins walking toward the hotel.

Laura helps me up, and then she follows Alexis.

I see the van come around the corner toward us. I watch in disbelief as it stops and the men shove both girls in the van. I'm left standing there, unable to help them.

Could this night get any worse? I don't know what to do to help my friends.

I head up to our room to find the cocaine and any cash. Our room looks like a hurricane hit it. There's no money and no cocaine. I quickly look in the bottom drawer of the dresser. I had discovered that a piece of wood at the bottom was loose and had hidden my passport there. *Thank goodness, my passport is still here.*

I run down the back stairs to the lobby.

"What do I do now?" I yell.

The manager comes out. "How can I help?" he asks.

I tell him the whole story.

"One of your friends is at the police station," he says, showing no emotion.

"Thank you," I reply, and then sprint out the front door. The police station is not far from the hotel. I stand at the front door and question whether I should go in, knowing that Mexican jails are notorious for injustice. I walk in hesitantly and see Arnie sitting on a metal chair.

"Arnie, what's going on?" I ask, out of breath.

"Oh, man, you're alive!" Arnie jumps up and hugs me.

"They took the girls!" I shout.

"No! What do we do?" he asks in disbelief. "Why did they kidnap you? Now the girls?"

"I have no idea. We just have to pray the girls are unharmed. Where's Ben?" I ask.

"Ben is being detained for running from the police," Arnie explains. "He told me he thinks the police are involved somehow."

We both just sit there in silence for several minutes.

"Here's what we do. We bail Ben out. Then we figure out how to find the girls," I state.

Arnie just nods. He offers the police all the money he has on him, and they reluctantly let Ben go. The three of us stand outside the jail.

Could the cops be involved? Is the manager an accomplice?

Arnie starts freaking out and throws up in the bushes. And Ben's so beat up by the cops that he's coughing and trying to catch his breath.

"Ben, why did you run away with the bag?" I ask him, now furious.

"Josh, I'm so sorry. I've been cheated out of what I've paid for before. I didn't want it to happen again, but I had no idea they would kidnap you, or Alexis and Laura!"

"We need to head back to the hotel," I tell both of them. I can't even look at Ben.

Arnie and Ben follow me in silence. The manager greets us as we enter the lobby.

"I know where they are," he says, as if he were relaying the time.

"Where?" Arnie exclaims.

At this point, the manager changes his story. "I will be right back," he says.

I'm so mad that I want to kill the assholes that took me at gunpoint. And now they have Alexis and Laura. I have to get it together, but all I can think about is Alexis or Laura being hurt, raped, or killed.

God, please tell me what to do next.

The manager comes back. "They just want their cocaine back and money."

"You said you knew where the girls were!" I exclaim.

"They've done this before, and they usually go back to Tequila," the manager continues.

"They 've done this before?" I scream at the manager. "Why didn't you tell me earlier when I told you what had happened?"

The manager says nothing, and I'm convinced that he's involved somehow.

"Well, we need to go back there, then," Arnie says.

"Hold up, they will be expecting that. We have to come up with a better plan," Ben states.

But we have no other plan. I'm still shaken up after having a gun pointed at my head. The girls must be terrified!

Just then, Ben's phone rings.

"Where are they?" Ben yells into the phone. "You can have the coke back. Just bring the girls to the hotel." He looks exhausted.

We have to pray that they will bring them back safe. Sitting in the lobby just waiting is the worst. Almost an hour later, Alexis walks through the front door. My heart sinks.

"Where's Laura?" I scream.

Alexis hugs Arnie and turns to me. "They have Laura in the van. They want you to bring out the coke."

"Why me? Why not Ben?" I swallow hard. "OK," I manage to say as fear runs up my spine. Ben hands me the bag.

The same dilapidated white van is parked out front.

The door slides open, and Laura screams, "Oh, Josh!"

"Bring the cocaine here," one guy says.

"Let her go, and I will walk toward you," I challenge him.

They release Laura, and she jumps out of the van. I walk toward them.

"Here." I hand them the same bag they gave us four hours earlier. The runt of the group snatches it and throws it in the van.

"Gringo," he says, laughing as he slams the van door shut.

They speed away. I turn around, and Laura runs toward me. She hugs me so hard and doesn't let go. We both cry. She tries to speak, but the words get caught in her throat.

"You're safe," I say, comforting her.

We stay there for several minutes. Alexis and Arnie run out of the hotel.

"Oh, thank God you're both safe," Alexis shouts.

Back in the hotel, we exchange glances. No one says anything for a long time.

"Wow, I can't believe we're all safe," Laura finally says. "I'm so thankful to be alive."

"Do you think we will be safe here tonight?" Alexis asks. "I can look for another hotel."

"Yes," I respond. "They got what they wanted," I offer as consolation. *But I don't know for sure. What if they come back?*

"Ben, how could you keep the cocaine, especially when they took Josh, Alexis, and me?" Laura asks.

"I'm so sorry." Ben puts his head down and starts to cry.

"We should all head to bed," Arnie adds. "We can look for a new place tomorrow."

Arnie, Ben, and I walk up the stairs to our room. We clean up the mess in silence.

I take off my clothes and put on a clean pair of shorts. I crawl into my bed.

All of us could have died tonight. How could Ben have been so selfish?

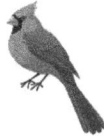

CHAPTER SIXTY-TWO

A Mother's Instinct

Maria

I wake up in a sweat. It's still dark outside. Something doesn't feel right in my gut.

Just then, Josh comes to mind.

God, please protect my son in Mexico.

I must have fallen back to sleep, because the sun is up now. I shower and get dressed and head downstairs to find Grant making breakfast for us.

"Hi, good morning," he says, and then gives me a kiss. "Did you sleep well?"

"Not sure. I woke up with a strange feeling about Josh around four o'clock this morning. I said a prayer for him and fell back asleep."

"What do you think the feeling was?" Grant asks.

"I think I'm just concerned about him flying back from Mexico."

"Flights are still continuing this week, so hopefully they will all fly home safe," he says to reassure me.

"I hope so," I whisper.

Grant hugs me. "Bye. See you after work."

Thankfully, the day goes fast, and tomorrow is Friday. Grant has been off today, and when I get home, he has made dinner for us. I really do love my generous husband. I change out of my dress and put on joggers and a comfy sweater. Pulling my phone out of my purse, I send Josh a quick text. *Hi, how are you? Your flight still scheduled for Saturday?*

I know he will respond, so I go downstairs to have dinner with Grant. The steak and potatoes are delicious. After dinner, I still have not heard from Josh.

"I think I'm going to bed early," I tell Grant.

"Sweetheart, he will be alright." Grant comes over to hug me.

"I know, I'm just really tired," I respond. "I love you."

"Love you, sleep well. I will be up soon," he replies.

Our love continues to provide hope and comfort for me.

It's several hours later, and Josh has not responded. *God, please protect Josh.*

I sleep terribly again; I keep waking up and looking at my phone to see if Josh has sent a text back. The morning comes too soon, and a hot shower does not help. Driving to work, I cry the whole way. I hide my phone in my drawer so I won't keep checking it.

After lunch, I open the drawer. Oh, thank goodness, Josh finally sent a text.

Hi, Mom. I'm good. Today is our last day here. Yes, my flight is still scheduled for tomorrow.

I breathe out in pure relief.

God, thank you for watching over my son.

The end of the day cannot come soon enough. I call Grant on the way home.

"I heard from Josh, and his flight is still leaving Mexico tomorrow."

"That's wonderful news. You on your way home?" he asks me.

"Yes, it is. I'm on my way home. See you soon."

I'm so relieved Josh sent me a text, but my "mom" intuition is telling me something is still not right. I will trust that God is with Josh, and that thought brings me peace.

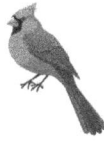

CHAPTER SIXTY-THREE

Last Day in Mexico

Josh

The sun wakes me up. It's our last day in Mexico. I feel happy and sad at the same time.

Last night comes back to me in a rush. *I was so scared. I'm thankful we're safe. We were there for one another; I know we will be friends for life.* I have come to realize that, even during very stressful situations, I have the courage and strength to get through things. And I can handle the times when anxiety and depression threaten to take over my mind.

I head downstairs, order a cup of coffee, and sit outside in the courtyard.

"Hi, good morning—you're up early today," Laura exclaims as she joins me outside. "Alexis and Arnie are looking for another hotel."

"Good morning. I hope they can find one, just for tonight."

We drink our coffee and silently agree not to talk about last night.

"We still have one more day," I remind Laura.

"Yes, you're right. What should we do today?" she asks.

"I say we make it another beach day," I suggest.

"That sounds perfect," she agrees.

"Hi, morning," Alexis says, joining us. "Arnie and I found another hotel."

"That's great. When can we check out of here?" Laura asks.

"Right away, and the new hotel can store our stuff until check-in this afternoon."

"Laura and I were talking about making it another beach day," I share with the group.

"Yeah, we were thinking the same thing," Arnie concurs.

"How about Alexis and I grab breakfast sandwiches, lunch meat, bread, and snacks?" Laura suggests. "Josh, you and Ben can get beverages. And, Arnie, can you get beach entertainment?"

"Sure thing," Arnie states.

We head upstairs to get our swimsuits on and pack our bags.

Ben is up when Arnie and I get to the room.

"Hey, Ben, we found a new hotel, so we're going to pack up our things and check out," Arnie tells him.

"Put your bathing suit on because we're going to the beach after," I add.

We meet in the lobby and check out of our respective rooms. Luckily, only the receptionist is working, and we don't have to see the awful manager.

After we drop off our bags at the new hotel, the girls head to the market. Ben, Arnie, and I head out to get beer, water, Frisbees, and a soccer ball.

Walking to the beach, I see a white van turning the corner. I freeze. *It's not them, but my heart is racing.*

Alexis and Laura are at the beach with the food when we get there.

We each spread out a towel, and we all sit for a moment in silence.

"I want to say I'm sorry again, for last night," Ben begins. "I never meant to put anyone in danger. I hope you can all forgive me."

"We forgive you, Ben," Alexis says, wiping away a tear.

Arnie pats Ben on the back, and I nod, taking in his apology.

Ben gets up and gathers several beer cans in his arms. He offers each of us a beer.

"A toast to an awesome week in Mexico with great friends." Ben raises his red Solo cup.

"Cheers," we all toast in unison. *We all know how lucky we are to be alive.*

"And cheers to us all being safe," Laura adds.

"Cheers," we all say again.

"How about a game of Frisbee?" Arnie asks.

"I'm going to sit this one out and work on my tan," Alexis says.

"I'll play," Laura says. "Josh and me against you and Ben."

"Oh, perfect. We're going to win," Ben yells.

"Don't get too cocky, Ben. I have a pretty good arm," Laura challenges.

Finishing my beer, I find the perfect spot to start our game.

"Laura, you're really good at this. But so is Arnie," Ben says.

Ben keeps missing the Frisbee and spews all kinds of profane language on the beach. "Ugh, I suck today. Alright, you won the first game. Rematch?"

"One more game," I agree.

Ben does better on the second game, but Laura and I still win. We all shake hands, although Ben is seriously pouting.

"We can play soccer later. I will win that," he says and heads to get another beer.

"Great game, Josh." Laura shakes my hand.

"You too," I return. "Last one in is a rotten egg." I tear off my T-shirt and run toward the water.

"Oh, I'm right behind you!" Laura shouts.

We're both laughing when we reach the water. It feels amazing. We hold hands and jump though the waves together. I can't stop smiling.

This is how life is meant to be, laughing and having fun. I want my life to be as happy as I have been this week. Well, except for last night.

Laura catches me looking at her, and she blows me a kiss. Back on the beach, we both fall asleep on our towels.

I wake up before Laura does. She is sleeping so peacefully. Then, she wakes up and catches me looking at her. She smiles and brushes her hair out of her eyes.

"Josh, thank you for such a great week."

"Well, we all pitched in," I say simply.

"I mean, thank you for letting me see the real you," Laura continues.

"You too," I reply, blushing.

Laura holds my hand. I enjoy just sitting next to her, watching the waves roll onto the shore.

"Who wants a sandwich?" Alexis asks.

"I do, thank you," Arnie answers.

"Me too," says Ben.

"I'll have one," I respond.

"I'll have one a little later." Laura holds on to my hand.

I don't let go of Laura's hand until Alexis hands me my sandwich. Ben passes beer around to everyone.

"Alexis and Laura, thank you for the sandwiches and snacks," Arnie says.

"And thank you, boys, for the beverages and games." Alexis continues to pass out the sandwiches.

"OK, now that our parents will be proud since we all have manners, who's ready for a soccer game?" Ben asks us all.

"I'll sit this one out," Arnie says.

CHAPTER SIXTY-THREE

So we play: Laura and me versus Alexis and Ben.

Alexis and Ben beat us.

"Good game," Laura announces, shaking hands with them.

It's getting late, so we start packing everything up. Walking back to our new hotel, I'm suddenly sad again. *I realize my sad thoughts are because I just don't want the week to end.*

"How about we get cleaned up and then meet in the lobby in an hour?" Alexis suggests.

We all agree and head upstairs. Once it's free, I spend a little longer than usual in the shower, just letting the hot water wash away the sand and grime and my sad thoughts.

Last night really frightened me. But it also showed me how important my life is.

I feel much better after my shower, and I put on my last clean shirt and shorts. After combing my hair, I head downstairs to meet everyone in the lobby.

"Time to make the most of our last night," Laura says to the group.

"Let's stay close. I'm still a little scared after last night," Alexis tells us. "We can go to our favorite mom-and-pop restaurant."

"Yeah, that's good," Ben continues. "Then we can hit a bar."

We head out to the restaurant. Once again, we order half the menu to share. I love the enchiladas, and I eat three right away. Ben orders us all tequila shots.

I sit and listen to everyone talk about our week. I'm enjoying being with my friends.

"Josh, you good?" Laura asks.

"Yeah, just a little tired. And you all have a lot to say," I respond.

"We always do," she says with her great smile.

We leave the restaurant stuffed and walk around a bit before heading to the bar.

I keep looking over my shoulder, fearful I may see those awful guys again.

"Let's go in here, they have the best local beer," Arnie suggests.

"Great idea," Alexis responds.

I feel relief after we get settled at our table and off the street.

After several rounds and much laughter, we start walking back to the hotel. I hear a loud noise. Pop. Pop. Pop. I look around, thinking the men in the white van are back.

I see kids shooting off bottle rockets. *I'm still shaken up after last night.*

We keep walking. *I feel calmer with my friends.*

"Our flight is still scheduled for tomorrow," Alexis says when we're back at the hotel.

"That's good. So many flights are being canceled because of this virus," Arnie adds.

"I really had a great time with all of you," I tell my wonderful friends.

Hugs for the girls, and then we all head upstairs.

I quickly brush my teeth and add the last few items to my suitcase.

In bed, I smile to myself.

Sleep comes quickly, but so does the morning. We grab our suitcases and go to meet the girls. They're already downstairs, and the Uber is on its way. We pile our stuff and ourselves into the Uber van and head to the airport. It looks like something from a movie. All the airport workers have masks on, and people look panicked.

"Our flight's still on time. Let's get through security." Alexis leads the way.

The wait in the security line is long; I'm glad we got here early. We finally make it through security and find our gate. Arnie and I grab biscuits and coffee for all of us. There are many announcements about canceled flights, but our flight is still scheduled to leave on time. Finally, they announce for us to board. I think we all let out a sigh of relief when the plane finally takes off.

I wake up just in time to see the Golden Gate Bridge come into view. We sit on the tarmac in a line of planes since many planes have been diverted to this airport.

"Maybe we should have stayed in Mexico. It seems crazy here in the United States." Ben looks concerned.

Finally, we are given the go-ahead to go to our gate. After collecting our luggage and having a quick bathroom break, we're ready to get one last Uber van to take us home. We're all exhausted and happy to be home. I put my suitcase in the corner of my room and head to take a shower. When I finish, I find Alexis and Arnie watching the news in the living room.

"They're saying that the virus is spreading quickly. They're starting to shut down airports, train stations, and many businesses downtown," Arnie explains.

"Looks like we just made it home in time," I respond.

"We sure did," Alexis says. "Anyone want grilled cheese?"

"Yes," Ben, Arnie, and I say in unison. Alexis heads to the kitchen and makes a sandwich for each of us. It's the best grilled cheese I've ever tasted.

None of us mention the cocaine and kidnappings. I think we just want to have a few normal days, and then we can discuss it. After helping Alexis clean the dishes, I head to my room. I'm so tired, I climb into my bed and close my eyes.

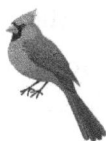

CHAPTER SIXTY-FOUR

Pandemic's Grip

Josh

For three days, I sleep day and night. I feel so terrible, I'm convinced I have the flu. And Alexis, Arnie, and Laura are feeling bad too. I drag myself out of bed and into the shower. As I stand there with the hot water hitting my skin, I start to feel a little better.

I find one clean pair of pants and a sweater. I will definitely have to do the wash that's still piled up on the floor next to my suitcase.

In the kitchen, I forage for food in the pantry. All I can find is cereal, and I'm thankful it's Cinnamon Toast Crunch. I pour some into a bowl. I don't even add milk. I turn on the TV, and every channel has the same news, discussing the virus.

Could I have contracted this virus? I have most of the symptoms they're talking about.

I hate being sick, and this is the worst I have felt physically in a long time.

I turn off the TV and head outside to our back porch to get some fresh air. Laura's outside, having a cup of coffee.

"Hi, Josh, how you feeling?" she asks.

"I'm finally feeling better. How about you?" I ask her.

"I felt bad the first two days we were back. I feel much better today. Do you think we had that virus?" Laura questions.

"Not sure. I did just hear them talking about it again on the TV," I respond.

"Well, I just found out we're in quarantine here. School will be online the rest of the semester." Laura looks concerned.

"Wow, do the others know?" I ask her.

"Alexis and Arnie do. Ben's still at his parents' house."

"Arnie said he's starting to feel better too," I add.

We sit in silence for several minutes.

"Laura, I had fun in Mexico," I say, wanting to say more about us.

"Me too," Laura shares. "We are friends, right?"

"Yes, we are." I am relieved. "Laura, I do like you, but I need to focus on me."

"Josh, our friendship means so much to me."

"Me too." I reach out to touch her hand.

We didn't need to say it, but I'm glad we cleared the air.

"We need to make a grocery list and go to the store." Laura changes the conversation.

"Yes, we definitely do—this cereal is stale," I say, pointing to my bowl.

As Laura and I head out to the store, we notice how deserted the streets are in San Francisco. It's really eerie, and several of the stores have been vandalized. *I feel like we are in some kind of apocalyptic movie.*

Many of the shelves in the grocery store are empty, but we manage to get eggs, lunch meat, cheese, a loaf of bread, milk, and orange juice, as well as dinner for the next few nights.

For weeks, we have food delivered from the grocery stores. We get takeout sometimes too. Occasionally, we take walks, wearing masks just to get out of the house. I'm so unmotivated taking classes online, and my grades are suffering.

My depression is back, and so is the anxiety. I'm feeling emotionally and mentally drained. *Being isolated and not being able to go to class has been really hard on me. I'm thankful I am with friends. Being alone would have been awful. Being in lockdown magnifies my depression.*

I email the school counselor to discuss my grades and the option to drop two of my classes. I share that I'm feeling depressed and that my schoolwork is too much with my classes being online.

One day, when I venture out to take a walk, I have a panic attack.

I call Mom. "Mom, I think I am having an attack. I can't breathe well and—"

"Josh, breathe in—one, two, three, four. And breathe out—four, three, two, one." Mom repeats this with me several times.

She stays with me on the phone and waits for me to feel better.

"I feel a little better," I share with her. I sit down on a bench in the park.

"I'm glad the breathing helped. You can always go to urgent care if the attack returns," Mom reminds me. "And of course, you can always call me."

"Mom, I've been even more anxious being in quarantine. Thanks for helping me today."

"I love you. I will call you to tomorrow to see how you're feeling."

"OK. Love you, Mom."

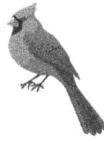

CHAPTER SIXTY-FIVE

Before the Storm

So, before you go
Was there something I could've said to make your heart beat better?
If only I'd have known you had a storm to weather
—"Before You Go," Lewis Capaldi

Maria

Heading to the airport, I'm thankful that Josh was able to get a flight to Charleston. After a month of being stuck in his apartment during quarantine in San Francisco, he decided to come home. I'm so excited to see him. When I park in the cell phone pickup area at the airport, I send him a quick text.

Hi, I'm here. Let me know when you're getting your bag at baggage claim.

Will do. We just landed, Josh responds.

Several restaurants have just reopened in Charleston. I search for one that has outdoor seating. Luckily, I find one restaurant with outdoor seating under a covered roof. It's supposed to start raining soon.

Just then Josh sends me a text. *I just got my bag.*

I will be right there, I text back.

I pull up and notice how skinny Josh is. *Has he been eating? Is he depressed? He must be. Being in quarantine, I'm starting to feel very depressed.*

I jump out of the car and give him a big hug.

"I'm happy to see you!" I help him get his bags in the trunk. "How was your flight?"

"It was fine. I slept some." Josh sounds exhausted.

"Are you hungry? Would you like to stop to get lunch?" I ask him, hoping he will agree.

"Yes, that would be great."

We're there in ten minutes, and I find a place to park. The hostess and server are both wearing masks. We wear our masks to the table. There's a storm coming, but I'm hopeful that we can eat before it arrives. Josh is quiet at first.

"So, tell me how school has been the last two months," I say, trying to break the ice.

"I was overwhelmed, and I dropped two classes. I was taking too many classes, and switching to online made it even more difficult. And my depression is back."

The storm moves in fast. The sky darkens, and rain starts to pelt the tin roof.

My heart sinks, hearing that Josh is depressed again. *How will he weather his mental health battle, being isolated and leaving his friends and his school?*

"I'm so sorry you're feeling depressed again. I can only imagine how hard it was to do your schoolwork online when you're used to seeing the professors and having hands-on instruction. How do you think you did in your exams?" I question him.

"I have no idea. I'm just glad it's over." Josh is quiet again. "I already miss my friends." He looks up, and I see tears fill his eyes.

"I know you do. Do you think you can room again next year?" I hesitantly ask.

"I'm not going back." Josh looks back down at his hands.

My heart sinks for my son. *He's worked so hard. This is so unfair after how hard he has fought to battle his anxiety and depression and after he went across the country for his education.*

"I'm proud of you for having the courage to go to California and take classes there this past year," I sincerely share with him.

"Thank you, Mom. I know I should've talked to you and Dad about my decision."

"Your dad and I will support you with any decision you make," I tell him.

"I know, and I appreciate that," Josh says, then hesitates. "First, I will have to deal with my depression. I just want to be healthy. And be happy."

"Let's call your psychiatrist and make an appointment." I look at him.

"Yes. And can I move in with you, Mom?" Josh asks me.

"Of course you can." I reach out to hold his hand.

I smile at my strong, handsome son. That has been my wish for him too—for him to be healthy and happy.

I pray that Josh finishes college and gets a great job he loves. I pray he finds his soulmate and has love in his life. I pray he understands that, in life, there may be pain, but he can feel the pain and then the joy. And I pray he will be free of the cage of depression that has held him captive.

I know Josh is fortunate to have us as loving parents who continuously love and support him as he fights his battles of depression and mental illness. Our society has very little understanding of mental illness. Many healthcare facilities are not equipped to help the mentally ill.

I know Josh knows we love him and are always here for him. And I pray he knows that he has everything he needs inside himself to face anything. I want Josh to live his life fully, enjoying all of God's blessings.

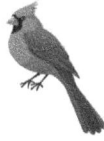

CHAPTER SIXTY-SIX

The Last Day

Maria

Josh lived with me for a year, and then he decided he wanted his own apartment. He had received his associate degree in computer sciences and accepted a remote position with a great company. He was seeing his high school friends and dating some. He even adopted two female kittens, sisters, whom he named Adriana and Karine. After nine months living on his own, he took a turn for the worse—he would walk for hours and barely eat. Josh told me that he wanted to leave Charleston and live with his dad, who had just built a new home in the mountains of Georgia.

I really thought this change would help Josh. And that he and Aaron could bond again.

I drove up separately to help Josh bring all his things and his kittens to his dad's new home.

Josh has been at his dad's place for several weeks when I call him on Thanksgiving Day. "Hi, Josh, Happy Thanksgiving. How's it going living with your dad?" I ask him.

"Hi, Mom. It's been good. I've been helping Dad put up the fence in the backyard," Josh replies.

"How have you been feeling?" I ask.

"Much better, Mom. Enjoy your Thanksgiving," he says quickly.

"You too. I love you." I wait for his response, but the line goes silent. Josh has hung up the phone.

Why was Josh so short with his response? I feel like he is keeping something from me.

I finish packing that night, as Grant and I are heading to Los Angeles for his very belated fiftieth birthday trip. Arriving in California the next day, we start our vacation in Santa Monica. In Los Angeles, we visit the television studios and go to a Los Angeles Chargers game.

On Monday, we drive from Los Angeles to Phoenix, Arizona. I'm so happy to attend an event hosted by my favorite mentor the next day. Very early in the morning, Grant drops me off at the front door of a beautiful mansion. I am greeted warmly and led to the sunroom for breakfast. Eating some berries and yogurt, I step out into the sunny backyard.

I just can't believe I'm here. I feel the sun on my face. I feel such peace and love, and I'm so excited for the event to begin. It's wonderful to be with these elegant women.

As we break for lunch, I open my phone to see I've missed several calls from Aaron. I call him back, and he starts yelling into the phone.

"Maria, Josh is gone! I went to the post office to mail one of my wooden tables. When I came back, I didn't see him in his room. I searched inside and then outside."

Aaron pauses. *The silence is too much.* Every terrible thought crosses my mind.

"Maria, Josh hanged himself." Aaron barely speaks above a whisper.

I drop my phone and fall to the floor.

I can feel the cold tile floor beneath me, but I don't feel like it's holding me ...

I feel like I'm falling ...

I try to breathe. I can barely get the air in and out. I start sobbing uncontrollably.

I can't stop.

I wail, and then gasp for air. A few of the ladies gather around me to offer comfort. They tell me they've called Grant to come to pick me up. I continue sobbing.

I remember being hugged by my mentor and her son. I remember Grant's arms around me as I stumble to the car.

Then I feel numb. All the way back to the hotel, I stare out the car window at the barren Arizona desert.

Grant helps me out of the car and up the stairs to our hotel room. I go out to the balcony and stare at the empty playground in the middle of the courtyard.

I remember Josh playing at the playground near our house when he was little.

I can't believe my little boy is gone.

Now I feel everything—anger toward God, anger toward the doctors and therapists who couldn't help Josh, and anger at depression, the awful monster that killed my son! Then the sadness returns.

I start crying again and I can't stop—the sadness is excruciating.

I don't know how long I have been sitting on the balcony.

I know I have to let Curt and Audra and AJ know—but how do I tell them their brother is gone?

When I call Audra, her dad has already talked to her, and she is crying hysterically. Luckily, her best friends are driving to our house to be with her. Next, I call AJ; he's in shock and doesn't talk much. Then I call Curt—he's quiet at first. Then he's upset that AJ will not drive the three hours to be with their dad.

Grant reaches out to my friends and the rest of my family.

"Josh, I thought you were feeling better. Why did you take your life?" I whisper into the suffocating air.

Silence.

Grant comes to hug me again. He holds me and doesn't let go.

"Maria, you need to eat something," he whispers to me.

"I'm not hungry," I respond flatly.

After he asks me a few more times, I agree to go with him to eat at a restaurant nearby. It's an Italian restaurant, and the menu does look good.

I get up to go to the bathroom to wash my hands. I look at my face in the mirror.

I look past my tearstained face and into my eyes. I see Josh's eyes looking back at me.

I start crying again.

After dinner, Grant suggests we drive to an overlook to watch the sunset from the mountain.

We get out of the car and walk to the overlook. The sky is beautiful—orange and mauve and pink. I feel the warm desert breeze envelop me.

Normally, I love watching the sunset. But my joy is gone.

Just then I can hear in my head words that I didn't think …

Mom, I know it's hard to understand. It was too painful. I tried for so long. I never felt better.

CHAPTER SIXTY-SIX

Josh, is that you? I question him in my mind. *I miss you so much already!*

It's me, Mom. I love you and Dad, and Curt, Audra, and AJ.

"Why, Josh, why?" I say out loud. Grant grabs my hand.

Mom, just know that I am happy. And I'm at peace now.

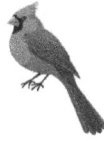

CHAPTER SIXTY-SEVEN

Reflections from Beyond

I faced it all, and I stood tall ...
I've loved, I've laughed and cried ...
I've had my fill, my share of losing ...
For what is a man, what has he got?
If not himself ...
The record shows I took the blows
And did it my way
—"My Way," Frank Sinatra

Josh

Later that night, I pick up the journal Mom gave me years ago. For a moment, I just hold it, letting the weight of it settle in my hands. Finally, I open to the first page and begin to write.

God, I believe you love me and are always there for me. Thank you for my family and my friends, who unconditionally love me. I will continue to ask for help, especially with depression, anxiety, or any mental health issue. It's my prayer that more people ask for help and that our world becomes more empathetic and understanding of mental illness.

I take a deep breath, letting the words sink into my being. This journal entry isn't just a note to God or myself—it feels like a step forward, a way to honor the journey I've been on and the people who have been by my side.

I pray for a world where no one feels ashamed to reach out for help, where conversations about mental health are met with understanding instead of judgment. I hope that we can all learn to be more compassionate toward others—and ourselves—and that we recognize the courage it takes to keep going, no matter how unbelievably hard it is.

Closing the journal, I press it against my chest. I feel the weight of everything I've been through, but I also feel a sense of peace, a sense of hope. I know that healing isn't perfect or even easy, but it's possible. *God, thank you for reminding me that I'm not alone.*

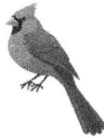

A flock of birds hovering above ...

That's how you think of love ...

I always look up to the sky and pray before the dawn ...

Maybe one day I'll fly next to you ...

Maybe one day I can fly with you

"Fly On" —Coldplay

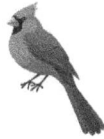

ACKNOWLEDGMENTS

God, thank you for the gift of my son Jonathan, who is with you now. Thank you for all of my children and for my husband, my family, and my friends.

Jonathan, my amazing, courageous son. Thank you for choosing me to be your mom. I love you, and I am forever blessed.

Chris, my oldest son, I love you. You trusted yourself to take a big leap to live your desires and move across the world. You inspire me every day to live my life to the fullest.

Allison, my beautiful daughter, I love you. You bring such joy to my life. I continue to cheer you on to fully live your dreams.

Anderson, my youngest son, you've shown me the strength of independence. My hope for you is to pursue your passionate dreams. I love you, and I'm here for you always.

Andy, we have loved our children with consistency and strength. I know Jonathan is with us all every day.

Gary, my beloved, thank you for loving me through it all. I love you and know you will always be by my side.

Mom, you have always been my number one cheerleader. Thank you for your love and support always.

Dad, I love you. Thank you for giving me the gift of persistence and for teaching me to never give up on my dreams.

Mindy, you and I share a heartfelt friendship of faith, supporting and loving our sons as they battled mental illness. I love you, my dear friend.

Jenny and Tara, I am forever grateful for your beautiful mentorship of light and love for me always.

My Forbes Books team—Suzanna, Katie, Adam, Alison, Annie, David, Elizabeth, Megan, and Olivia—I'm thankful for your hours of devotion to bring this book to life.

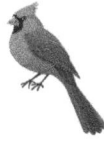

ABOUT THE AUTHOR

Dawn Lohr is a devoted mother of four grown children and a graduate of Loyola University in Maryland, where she earned a degree in marketing. With a passion for entrepreneurial ventures, Dawn has ventured into successful businesses and achieved remarkable success in her home-based business, which allowed her to expand and grow while raising her family. No matter what she is doing, she always showcases her knack for innovation and growth. Dawn is continually seeking new avenues for expansion and development. Her most profound journey, however, has been her transition into speaking and authorship, marked by the release of this deeply moving and inspirational book dedicated to her son Jon, whom she tragically lost to suicide in 2023.

As a dynamic and powerful speaker, Dawn captivates audiences with her passionate and open-hearted approach. Her resilience and strength are evident as she shares her personal journey through the complexities of mental health, the challenges of balancing life's demands, and the heart-wrenching moment she learned, while attending a conference, of her son's passing. Through her unimaginable grief, Dawn has discovered a wellspring of inspiring stories and events, offering hope and healing to others. Her profound connection with Jon's spirit serves as a poignant reminder of the eternal bonds we share with our loved ones, guiding us through life's most challenging moments with grace and love.

—Jenny Aiello,
Life development coach

www.ingramcontent.com/pod-product-compliance
Lightning Source LLC
Chambersburg PA
CBHW020453100426

42813CB00031B/3354/J